“Take time by the forelock”:

The Letters of Anthony Fothergill to James Woodforde

1789–1813

(*Medical History*, Supplement No. 17)

"Take time by the forelock":

The Letters of Anthony Fothergill to James Woodforde

1789–1813

edited by

CHRISTOPHER LAWRENCE, PAUL LUCIER
AND CHRISTOPHER C. BOOTH

(*Medical History*, Supplement No. 17)

London
Wellcome Institute for the History of Medicine
1997

ISBN 0 85484 066 4

Supplements to *Medical History* may be obtained by post from Professional and Scientific Publications, BMA House, Tavistock Square, London WC1H 9JR.

Contents

Preface

This project began when Christopher C. Booth offered the letters to Christopher Lawrence for co-editing. In fact the bulk of the editorial work was shared by Christopher Lawrence and Paul Lucier who are grateful to Sir Christopher for his initial kind offer. They are also grateful for his biographies of Anthony Fothergill and James Woodforde in the Introduction, and his support and input in all sorts of ways.

Acknowledgements

We are grateful to the American Philosophical Society for permission to publish the letters and to Whitfield Bell Jr. for his assistance in this and other matters. Thanks go to Nat Booth for translating, correcting and tracking down the Latin quotations and to Melvin Earles for his help in deciphering the prescriptions. We are grateful to the Wellcome Trust for the grant that made Paul Lucier's share of the editing possible.

Introduction

In the Library of the American Philosophical Society at Philadelphia there is a letterbook. It is titled, in the same hand as the letters, 'A collection of Letters from Dr A. Fothergill to J. Woodforde M.D.'.[1] The letters of Anthony Fothergill (1737–1813) to James Woodforde (1771–1837) cover the period 1789–1813. At the time the correspondence commenced Fothergill was a distinguished physician practising in Bath and Woodforde was apprentice to two surgeon-apothecaries in the West Country. Fothergill became Woodforde's patron and the letters record Fothergill's ongoing advice, material assistance and attempts to use his influence on Woodforde's behalf until Fothergill's death shortly after the last letter. Woodforde served his apprenticeship between 1786–1791 and then went to study at the Edinburgh medical school. Three years later, in 1794, he qualified as an MD. He then returned to the West Country and endeavoured to establish himself in practice as a physician.

The letters are a rich source of information for the student of Georgian social life, for they are not confined to technical medical issues. They discuss, for example, the Bath season, the Napoleonic Wars, American affairs, the cost of living and the vagaries of travel and those of the post. For the medical historian in particular, however, the letters are a gold mine. Fothergill's advice to Woodforde as a student included a comprehensive account of the books he considered the aspiring physician should read. It covered the order in which he thought medical lectures should be attended and an evaluation of the various Edinburgh professors. Fothergill also guided Woodforde on how to conduct himself so as to make the best impression on his teachers. Fothergill's reflections on Woodforde's Edinburgh experiences shed much light on student life in Edinburgh. After Woodforde's qualification, the letters are full of remarks on how to construct a successful medical career. The politics of hospital appointments, the challenge of the surgeon-apothecary to the physician and the importance of midwifery, all make their appearance. The letters are crammed with details of the books exchanged between the correspondents and their discussion of new medical theories, such as those of John Brown and Benjamin Rush. Their increasing exchange of journals would seem to be a measure of the rising importance of periodical literature in science and medicine in this period.[2] Actual medical practice figures large too. There are detailed accounts of patients, their illnesses and prescriptions. Significantly, on occasion, physical examination of patients makes an appearance (letters **54** and **71**). The historian of science will find pertinent material here too. Natural philosophical texts, itinerant lecturing, the chemical revolution and electricity are all discussed.

Anthony Fothergill MD

Anthony Fothergill (1737–1813) lived for much of his life in the shadow of his more distinguished namesake, Dr John Fothergill (1712–1780). It was to John Fothergill, the famous Quaker physician of eighteenth-century London, that Anthony referred in the first letter in this series, in which he disclaimed "the encomiums which justly belong to my late

[1] Anthony Fothergill, Letters to J. Woodforde. A Letterbook, 1 volume, 258 pp. B F823, Film 1411. American Philosophical Society, Philadelphia.

[2] Susan C. Lawrence, *Charitable knowledge: hospital pupils and practitioners in eighteenth-century London*, Cambridge University Press, 1996.

illustrious and ever to be revered namesake, whose character you wish to emulate . . ." (letter **1**). Anthony Fothergill was more than twenty years younger than John. Although they both hailed from the north of England and received their education at the same school at Sedbergh, they were not relations. John Fothergill came from a small valley branching off Wensleydale in north Yorkshire, from a family that had been strict Quakers for four generations.[3] Anthony Fothergill came from Ravenstonedale in Westmorland and, even though they were only twenty-five miles apart, the families cannot be positively connected. The Westmorland Fothergills were an Anglican conformist family which produced several men of learning and ability.[4] Thomas Fothergill was Master of St John's College, Cambridge, in the mid-seventeenth century and, later, George Fothergill was principal of St Edmund Hall. His brother Thomas was Provost of Queen's College, Oxford, from 1767 until his death in 1796. Anthony Fothergill came from a more obscure branch of this family. His father Anthony, who was probably a farmer, married Frances Bainbridge in 1735. They lived in a small hamlet called Murthwaite, now no more than a few uninhabited farm buildings which can be reached only by a track across the fields. Here their son Anthony was born and he was christened in Ravenstonedale Church on 12 March 1736/7.[5]

Anthony was educated at nearby Sedbergh School where he would have learnt the classical languages then necessary for entry into the study of medicine. In 1755, he was apprenticed to his maternal cousin, John Drake Bainbridge,[6] a well-known apothecary, an influential figure in Durham who became mayor of the city six times between 1761 and 1794. Anthony Fothergill remained with him for five years and then went to Edinburgh as a medical student. He joined the prestigious Royal Medical Society (RMS) in 1761 and graduated MD in 1763 with a thesis on intermittent fever. The thesis was dedicated to his teacher, William Cullen, and to Sir Ralph Milbanke.[7] Sir Ralph was the fifth baronet and a landowner in Yorkshire and Durham. He had been member of parliament for Scarborough from 1754 to 1761 but by 1763 he was the member for the large constituency of Richmond, Yorkshire, which still extends as far as the old Westmorland border. Sir Ralph was no rural dullard. His family had important connections. His daughter Elizabeth became the first Lady Melbourne, the mother of Queen Victoria's first prime minister.[8] His granddaughter, Anne Isabella Milbanke, had the misfortune to marry the wayward Lord Byron.[9] Sir Ralph and Anthony Fothergill's master, John Bainbridge, were also connected by marriage. It is therefore reasonable to conclude that Sir Ralph had contributed to Anthony's education in Edinburgh, just as Anthony himself was to do later for James Woodforde.

Soon after his graduation, the young Anthony Fothergill met John Fothergill in London and on his counsel settled in Northampton as a physician in 1764. He was appointed

[3] See R. H. Fox, *Dr John Fothergill and his friends: chapters in eighteenth-century life*, London, Macmillan, 1919. B. C. Corner and C. C. Booth, *Chain of Friendship. Letters of Dr John Fothergill of London, 1735–1780*, Cambridge, Massachusetts, Harvard University Press, 1971.

[4] C. Thornton and F. MacLaughlan, *The Fothergills of Ravenstonedale: their lives and their letters*, London, Heinemann, 1905.

[5] Parish Register, Ravenstonedale Church. Copy at the Society of Genealogists.

[6] A detailed genealogy of the Fothergill and Bainbridge families has been prepared by Dr G. C. R Morris of Orpington, Kent. Dr Morris is a lineal descendant of John Drake Bainbridge.

[7] Sir Ralph Milbanke, 5th Bt (1725–1798) was the son of the 4th Baronet through his second marriage to Ann Delaval.

[8] Elizabeth Milbanke (1749–1818) married Viscount Melbourne on 13 April 1769. Her son William Lamb, later Viscount Melbourne, was born on 15 March 1779.

[9] Anne Isabella Milbanke (1792–1860) married Lord Byron on 2 January 1815.

physician to the General Infirmary in Northampton in December of that year but seems to have met with unexpected difficulties. Dr John wrote encouragingly to him from London: "Depend more on propriety of conduct than on recommendations, though these ought not to be neglected. Have patience, be firm".[10] Throughout his years in Northampton, Anthony corresponded with John and some of this correspondence appears in J. C. Lettsom's memoir of John Fothergill, published after his death from prostatic obstruction in 1780.[11] It was a task that Lettsom, John's protégé, was well able to undertake. Anthony Fothergill was later to hope that Lettsom would do the same for his own memory.

In 1778, Anthony was elected to the Royal Society, having been proposed as a "gentleman well versed in mathematics, natural philosophy and the learned languages".[12] John Fothergill was his second sponsor, William Hunter the third, indicating the high regard in which he had now come to be held. The following year he became a Licentiate of the Royal College of Physicians,[13] an essential step if he was to practise as a prominent mainstream physician in London. In 1781, he moved to London in an attempt to fill his distinguished namesake's place. He appears to have lived for a while in the doctor's house in Harpur Street, presided over by John's formidable Quaker sister Ann.[14] He did not, however, prosper and it was Lettsom who was to inherit John's position in London medicine.

The next year, Anthony Fothergill moved to Bath where he was to spend the most fruitful years of his career. He lived at No. 9, Walcot Parade, a terrace of houses on the London road.[15] He became an active member of the Medical Society of London, which had been founded by Lettsom in 1773, contributing papers on influenza, consumption and the treatment of epilepsy. But his main interest was in the fledgling Royal Humane Society, founded by William Hawes and Thomas Coggan in 1774.[16] The Society was particularly concerned with the resuscitation of persons apparently dead from drowning. The means of restoring animation were Anthony Fothergill's particular interest. The topic was the source of much correspondence between Fothergill and Woodforde and was to be the subject of the latter's MD thesis in Edinburgh when he submitted it in 1794. That same year, Anthony Fothergill was awarded a gold medal by the Royal Humane Society for an essay on the subject.[17] Whilst in Bath, he wrote on lead poisoning, rabies, and the abuse of spirituous liquors. He published a tract on the use of the Cheltenham waters in 1788[18] and in 1792 he had the distinction, along with Lettsom, of being elected a foreign member of the American Philosophical Society.[19]

[10] R. H. Fox, op. cit., note 3 above, pp. 131–3.

[11] J. C. Lettsom, *The works of John Fothergill M.D. with some account of his life*, London, C. Dilly, 1783–84.

[12] Archives of the Royal Society, London.

[13] Annals of the Royal College of Physicians of London (1779), XIV, 112, 113 and 115.

[14] C. C. Booth, 'Ann Fothergill, the Mistress of Harpur Street', *Proceedings of the American Philosophical Society*, 1978, **122**: 340–54.

[15] Dr Anthony Fothergill's residence at 9, Walcot Parade is attested by street records of the City of Bath between 1784 and 1804, preserved in the Bath Public Library.

[16] P. J. Bishop, *A short history of the Royal Humane Society*, London, The Royal Humane Society, 1974.

[17] A. Fothergill, *A new inquiry into the suspension of vital action in cases of drowning and suffocation*, London, C. Dilly and Bath, R. Cruttwell, 1795.

[18] Anthony Fothergill's publications include: *An essay on the abuse of spirituous liquors*, Bath, R. Cruttwell, 1796. *A new experimental inquiry into the nature and qualities of the Cheltenham water*, Bath, R. Cruttwell, 1788. *Caution to the head of families, in three essays: (i) On cyder wine. (ii) On the poison of lead. (iii) On the poison of copper*, Bath, R. Cruttwell and London, C. Dilly, 1790. *On the nature of the disease produced by the bite of a mad dog*, Bath, R. Cruttwell, 1799.

In 1803, at the age of sixty-six, he decided, for health reasons (letter **82**), to give up what had become a highly successful practice as a physician and move to Pennsylvania. He travelled to Bristol to take ship for Philadelphia and arrived in the autumn, taking lodgings in Walnut Street. In Philadelphia he played an active role in the affairs of the American Philosophical Society, contributing on Bills of Mortality for the United States, "ice islands", population and on the cold in Northampton in 1776. He was a member of committees commenting on work submitted for publication by the Society and in 1804 he produced an almost skittish account of the virtues of the common hop, arguing that "the celebrated Nectar of the Heathenish gods, which they were said to have quaffed very freely to render themselves immortal, was none other than fine ale well hopped . . .". At the same time he made exhaustive daily observations on the weather, wind and temperature and wrote extensively on the population, longevity and diseases of Philadelphia. The work was never published, but the manuscript, a testament to the fertility of its author's mind, is preserved in the library of the American Philosophical Society.[20] A copy was sent to Sir Joseph Banks, President of the Royal Society in London.

Anthony Fothergill seems to have enjoyed an active social life in Philadelphia. He met distinguished medical men, among them John Morgan,[21] founder of the first medical school in the United States, and dined with him. He also visited the President, Thomas Jefferson, in Washington in 1804. He may have become acquainted with Jefferson through the Philosophical Society, for he was not only President of the United States but also President of the Society. Fothergill's letter of thanks following his visit, dated 8 June, is preserved in the Jefferson papers: "Dr Fothergill cannot leave the City of Washington without offering his grateful acknowledgements to the President of the US for his repeated civilities & kind hospitality, wishing him uninterrupted health & prosperity, begs leave to request his acceptance of these little tracts as a token of remembrance.[22] In 1812 the recurrence of war between Britain and the United States made his position in Philadelphia difficult and he decided to return to England. It was not to be for long. He must have had time to meet old friends from the Medical Society of London and he certainly met Lettsom again. But Fothergill was now an old man in his late seventies and he died at St George's Place on 11 May 1813.

His Will, a copy of which is preserved at the College of Physicians of Philadelphia,[23] was long and complicated, dealing with property on both sides of the Atlantic. He asked first that an oval marble tablet be placed in the Episcopal church in Philadelphia where he worshipped, to be inscribed with his name and the following alarming admonition: "Reader here make solemn pause. . . . Remember that on the present day hangs Eternity towards which thou art hastening . . .". He also asked that a pathetic funeral sermon be preached from the text: "Let us work while it is yet day for the night cometh when no

[19] Anthony Fothergill's acknowledgement of the receipt of his Diploma of Membership is given in a letter to George Turner of Bath, dated April 1792. MS autograph letter, Library of the American Philosophical Society.

[20] Fothergill's manuscripts on all these topics are preserved in the Library of the American Philosophical Society.

[21] John Morgan (1735–1789) played a major role in the foundation of the medical school in Philadelphia in 1765, after his return from studies in Europe. Whitfield J. Bell, *John Morgan, continental doctor*, Philadelphia, University of Pennsylvania Press, 1965.

[22] Anthony Fothergill to Thomas Jefferson. MS autograph letter addressed "To His Excellency the President of the United States. By favour of Mr Maddison". Jefferson Papers, Library of Congress, Washington, DC, USA.

[23] MS copy of the Will of the late Dr Anthony Fothergill. Library of the College of Physicians of Philadelphia.

man can work". This was given by the Reverend James Abercrombie and was later published in Philadelphia.[24] Fothergill left all his papers to Lettsom, together with £1,000 to be devoted to a "New and Elegant Edition of my Works . . .". But, because of difficulties over legacies to his Bainbridge relations, there were delays before the Will could be proved and Lettsom died in 1815 before he had received his legacy. Anthony Fothergill achieved a certain immortality by leaving £500 to the Medical Society of London to establish a medal in his memory. The Fothergillian Medal is awarded to this day. Among the many legacies that he made, there was one other to be noted. He left £100 to Dr Woodforde of Castle Cary.

James Woodforde MD

It was possibly through his extensive practice that Anthony Fothergill came to know the Woodforde family. At Bath there is little doubt that he was one of those fashionable doctors who attended the numerous upper-class invalids who came to take the waters of the spa. But, as his letters show, he also had a practice that extended widely throughout the surrounding countryside. The Woodforde family, living in or around Castle Cary, only twenty-five miles from Bath, were also sufficiently prosperous to consult one of the leading physicians in Bath.

James Woodforde, who belonged to this family, was born at Alhampton, Somerset, on 22 August 1771.[25] He was thought to be the seventh child of Heighes Woodforde (1725–1789), an unsuccessful lawyer, through his marriage to Anne Dorville. Heighes was the son of the Rector of Ansford, near Castle Cary, and the elder brother of Parson James Woodforde (1740–1803), the famous diarist. Parson Woodforde left Somerset to take up a living at Weston in Norfolk in 1774. He achieved literary immortality from the diary of everyday life that he kept from 1754 until 1803.[26] The diary records many of the activities of his family, including numerous convivial occasions with his brother Heighes. To the uninitiated therefore James Woodforde, future correspondent of Anthony Fothergill, would appear to have been a nephew of the diarist.

Yet all was not as it seemed.[27] Heighes Woodforde's union with Anne Dorville was a classic example of marrying in haste and repenting at leisure. Heighes, at the age of twenty-eight, eloped with Anne and they were married in the Savoy Chapel, London, on 17 December 1754. This clandestine ceremony was already illegal under the terms of Lord Hardwicke's Marriage Act, passed the previous year. It was presumably for this reason that the wedding was repeated in Anne's parish of Ditcheat on 22 January 1757, three months before the birth of their first child, a daughter, who was christened Anna Maria but who was later always known as "Nancy".

According to the Woodforde Family Book, Heighes Woodforde had a tempestuous relationship with his wife, Anne, an independent woman who had inherited property at

[24] James Abercrombie, *Funeral sermon on the importance and the improvement of time . . . in compliance with the desire expressed by the late Anthony Fothergill*, Philadelphia, James Maxwell, 1814.

[25] Parish Registers of Ditcheat, Somerset Record Office, Taunton.

[26] James Woodforde, *The diary of a country parson*, edited by John Beresford, 5 vols., Oxford, Clarendon Press, 1968.

[27] The details of the affairs of the Woodforde Family that follow have been taken from the Woodforde Family Book and have been kindly contributed by D. L. Winstanley Esq., editor of the *Quarterly journal of the Parson Woodforde Society*. The Society has one of two copies of the Woodforde Family Book.

Alhampton from her father. There were repeated rows and separations during the 1760s and in December 1770 the couple became totally estranged following a dramatic breakdown of their relationship. Heighes, then living at Ansford, sent his bed to Anne's house at Alhampton. Significantly Anne must have already been pregnant with her seventh child, James. There were stormy scenes and the bed was unceremoniously returned to Ansford. Heighes, like his bed, never returned to the marital home.

There is little doubt that Heighes Woodforde acknowledged the first four children born to the marriage as his own but in a draft of his Will dated 25 June 1783, he wrote of the three youngest children, Ralph, Francis and James, "I do solemnly declare and affirm that they are not to be mine".[28] The probated Will contains no such acknowledgement, possibly Woodforde wished to avoid the stigma of bastardising the children. So although James, future physician and correspondent of Dr Anthony Fothergill, was baptised a Woodforde, there is considerable doubt as to who his father was.

James Woodforde, born within months of the dramatic final breakdown of his parents' marriage, was brought up at his mother's house at Alhampton. We know nothing of James's education until he was apprenticed to two surgeon-apothecaries of Trowbridge, Wiltshire, in 1786. In 1788, when James was seventeen, Parson Woodforde wrote in his diary on 5 April that "Nancy", Heighes' eldest child then staying with him, had received a letter from "one Js Woodforde, who is apprenticed to an apothecary".[29] Parson Woodforde never referred to James as his nephew. In 1790, Parson Woodforde confided to his diary on 28 December that James's mother was "crazy and calls herself Lady Woodforde" but we have no independent corroboration of this observation.[30] There was no love lost between her and the Woodforde family. Parson Woodforde in his diary always referred to her as "Nancy's mother", whilst James, on the few occasions upon which he was taken note of, was the "son of Nancy's mother".

In 1791 James first went to Edinburgh as a student. The University records show that he matriculated for three successive sessions between 1791 and 1794 and that he spelt his name without an "e" (see below, p. xx, fn 49). As a medical student he appears to have been active in student affairs. Encouraged by Anthony Fothergill, he joined the prestigious RMS. Other societies with which he was involved included the Royal Physical Society and, curiously, the American Physical Society. He graduated MD in 1794, his thesis being entitled *De resuscitione submersorum.*[31] It was appropriately dedicated to his friend, mentor and financial supporter "Anthonio Fothergill M.D." and to "Gulielmo Hawes". As these letters show, it was Anthony Fothergill, friend and collaborator of William Hawes, who had suggested the subject.

Following his graduation, James Woodforde returned to his native Alhampton where at first he lived with his ageing mother. But he did not find it easy to obtain employment as a physician, even though Anthony Fothergill helped and advised him as much as he could. In that same year, 1794, his mother Anne Woodforde signed her Will, five years before her death.[32] In that document James is described as "of the City of Bristol, Doctor

[28] MS Will of Heighes Woodforde, dated 5 June 1783. New College archives No. 9537. By kind permission of the Warden and Scholars of New College, Oxford.

[29] Woodforde, op. cit., note 26 above, vol. 3, p.16.

[30] Ibid, p. 239.

[31] Jacobus Woodforde, *Tentamen medicum inaugurale de resuscitione submersorum*, Edinburgh, Balfour and Smellie, 1794.

of Physic". The Will also shows the close relationship that she had now developed with her son's mentor, for she chose Anthony Fothergill as one of her trustees. Anne died on 25 April 1799. The main provisions of her Will were aimed at the three children disowned by her husband, who had died ten years earlier and had already provided for the four older children whom he acknowledged as his own. Anne Woodforde's property did not pass directly to her children for she set up a Trust to administer her estate, with Anthony Fothergill and John Goldsmith as trustees. James, however, must now have benefited from the improvement in his circumstances and within two years he had chosen for himself a wife. He was married on 7 December 1801 to Juliana Clutterbuck, daughter of a solicitor of Marazion, Cornwall. There were five children of the marriage, all born within six years—Mary (b. 1802), James (b. 1804), Thomas (b. 1805), Juliana (b. 1806) and Henry (b.1807).[33]

Where James practised after his marriage is uncertain but at some time he settled at Ansford. He seems to have lived an uneventful life. He published in 1820 *A treatise on dyspepsia; or indigestion*[34] and a second edition appeared the following year. He apparently also published a brief work on an outbreak of typhus in the prison at Ilchester and gave evidence at the trial of the gaoler when he was prosecuted.[35] James Woodforde died at Castle Cary on the first day of 1837, the year of Queen Victoria's accession. A tablet commemorating his family is in Ansford Church. It reads: "In him were verified the words of Solomon. He who honoureth his Maker hath mercy on the poor".

James Woodforde was sufficiently prosperous to send two of his sons to study medicine in Edinburgh. His son James was a student between 1821 and 1825, when he graduated MD with a thesis entitled *De remediis purgantium*.[36] He dedicated his thesis to James Hamilton, Senior, the Edinburgh physician, to his father and to Henry Clutterbuck MD, who was his maternal uncle.[37] Clutterbuck was a prolific medical writer who had graduated MD in Glasgow in 1804. He later established himself as a leading physician and he was prominent in the affairs of the Medical Society of London. For many years he was physician to the General Dispensary in Aldersgate Street. It was presumably through his influence that the young James became a staff member there in 1828.[38] James junior was an able botanist, publishing a work on the flowers of Edinburgh in 1824.[39] There is a fleeting glimpse of him in the autobiographical writings of Dr John Mackenzie (1803–1886). Mackenzie records that whilst in Edinburgh in the 1820s, he made friends with

[32] 'The Will of Anne Woodforde', *Quarterly journal of the Parson Woodforde Society*, Winter 1994, pp. 28–30.

[33] Personal communication, D. L. Winstanley (see note 27 above).

[34] James Woodforde, *A treatise on dyspepsia; or indigestion*, Sherbourne, E. Penny, 1820.

[35] Personal Communication, D. L. Winstanley (see note 27 above). We have been unable to trace this work.

[36] Jacobus Woodforde, *De remediis purgantium*, Edinburgh, P. Neill, 1825.

[37] On James Hamilton see letter **86**, note 7. Henry Clutterbuck (1767–1856) was the fifth child of Thomas Clutterbuck of Marazion in Cornwall. He was the brother of James Woodforde Snr's wife. He became a member of the College of Surgeons in 1790 and worked first as a general practitioner in London. He then went to Glasgow, where he obtained his MD in 1804. Settling again in London, he built up a thriving clinical practice as well as excelling as a teacher. He founded and edited *The medical and chirurgical review*. His death in 1856 followed a street accident after he had attended a meeting at the Medical Society of London.

[38] The Aldersgate Dispensary Annual Report for 1937 lists all the physicians and surgeons to the Dispensary from 1770 and includes "James Woodforde M.D." as a physician in 1828. Information provided by Andrew Griffin, Trust Archivist, St Bartholomew's Hospital, London.

[39] James Woodforde Esq., *Catalogue of the indigenous phenogamic plants growing in the neighbourhood of Edinburgh; and of certain species of the class cryptogamia with reference to their*

"an English comrade named Woodford [*sic*], who was as devoted to flowers as I was" and he invited him to visit him at his home.[40] Soon after his graduation, James junior must have moved to London for he was elected to the Linnean Society in 1825, writing to acknowledge his election from an address in Fleet Street.[41] The letter is included as an appendix. James did not stay long in London for he joined the East India Company and in 1829 was an assistant surgeon in Madras. Like so many in colonial service in those days, he died young, succumbing at Guntur in 1838, at the age of thirty-four.

His younger brother Thomas also studied in Edinburgh, from 1822 until 1826, when he graduated MD with a thesis entitled *De mania*.[42] Like his brother, he dedicated the thesis to his father. Little is known of his subsequent career. According to the family records he practised at Taunton and died unmarried on 8 May 1843.

The Letters

The correspondence opens in August 1789, when Woodforde was apprentice to the surgeon-apothecaries William Palmer and Joseph Sylvester of Trowbridge, Wiltshire. Woodforde was already known to Fothergill, who wrote to him from Bath. Woodforde at this time was obviously uncertain as to whether to make his future as a physician, surgeon or apothecary. Fothergill offered to give Woodforde advice on the choice of books and the educational route he should follow whichever career he decided to take up. Already it was clear, at least to Fothergill, that if Woodforde elected to become a physician his best plan would be to study and graduate at Edinburgh. Shortly after the correspondence opened, Fothergill learned from Woodforde that he had opted to become a surgeon or surgeon-apothecary. Fothergill encouraged him to learn Latin, a little Greek, natural philosophy and chemistry, and recommended suitable texts. These things, according to the letters, Woodforde undertook. In 1790 Woodforde had decided to attend lectures at Edinburgh commencing in the academic year of 1791 when his apprenticeship would be finished. Fothergill then recounted to him some details of his own days in Edinburgh in the early 1760s.

By June 1790, Fothergill was recommending Woodforde to begin the study of physiology by reading the works of Albrecht von Haller. At the end of the year they were engaged in discussing quite detailed technical questions, such as the mode of action of digitalis (letter **10**), the status of Joseph Priestley's gas chemistry and the nature of animal heat (letter **11**). At this time too the first suggestion of the possible ill health of Woodforde's mother was raised (letter **10**), later to be a subject of considerable concern. During the first six months of 1791 a large number of books, mainly but not entirely medical, were exchanged between the correspondents. In the summer of that year Fothergill began to give Woodforde advice about how to proceed at the medical school (letter **15**). Woodforde was still intending to become a surgeon-apothecary (letter **16**) and, as Fothergill put it, considered his "views

---

location, Edinburgh, J. Carfrak and London, Longman, Hurst, Rees, Orme, Brown & Green, 1824.

[40] *Pigeon holes of memory. The life and times of Dr John Mackenzie (1803–1886)*, edited from his manuscript memoirs by Christina Byam Shaw, London, Constable, 1954, p. 119.

[41] The MS autograph letter is from 5 Bouverie Street and is dated "Monday Dec 13". James Woodforde laments his inability to attend the Linnean Society as arranged and asks that he may attend a future meeting so that "I can take my seat as a Fellow". It appears that he never did. Archives of the Linnean Society, Burlington House, London.

[42] Thomas Woodforde, *Dissertatio medica inauguralis de mania*, Edinburgh, P. Neill, 1826.

limited to surgery, pharmacy and midwifery". In the which case Fothergill advised that a single year in Edinburgh studying anatomy, attending the Royal Infirmary and taking classes in chemistry and materia medica would be sufficient. By August, Fothergill was giving Woodforde detailed advice about getting introductions to professors, finding lodgings, the sorts of clothes to wear and other things necessary for a profitable time at the medical school (letters **18**, **19**). In October 1791 Woodforde arrived in Edinburgh. He was still planning to stay only a year (letter **20**).

A Faculty of Medicine had been established in the University of Edinburgh in 1726. At the end of the century Edinburgh was the greatest medical school in Europe although its most glorious days were just over (it was shortly to be eclipsed by Paris). Its best years, not coincidentally, were those when Scotland's most famous literati also reigned: David Hume and Adam Smith for example.[43] At the end of the century the medical school was staffed by a number of capable but possibly lesser lights than those of the great days of the third quarter of the century. William Cullen, the internationally renowned professor of the practice of medicine, had died in 1790.[44] His successor, James Gregory, attained considerable fame but never quite the lustre of his predecessor. Joseph Black remained as professor of chemistry until his death in 1799, but his health was declining, and from about 1792 John Rotheram delivered a large part of the course, until Thomas Charles Hope was appointed conjoint professor with Black in 1796.[45] Alexander Monro *secundus*, professor of anatomy, was the only other internationally renowned figure. He continued to teach until 1798 when he was in his sixties, but the works for which he was famous had been published in the early and mid-1780s.[46] Andrew Duncan, the elder, professor of the Institutes of Medicine (later to be called physiology), and Francis Home, professor of materia medica, were highly respected teachers but not physicians of the stature of Cullen. The extra-mural school based mainly at and around the Royal College of Surgeons, however, and the students' RMS were flourishing.

Students of all sorts attended Edinburgh, notably surgeon-apothecaries who, after their apprenticeships, intended to add attendance at formal lectures to their credentials. There were also men intent on graduating MD. There were others who simply enrolled at various courses and then went off to practise or took the examination of the Royal College of Surgeons of Edinburgh or its London equivalent (not Royal until 1800).[47] Unlike Oxford and Cambridge, Edinburgh had no formal religious requirements and men of all denominations were to be found there. The school was a particular favourite with dissenters.

[43] For the school's greatest era see Christopher Lawrence, 'Ornate physicians and learned artisans: Edinburgh medical men, 1726–1776', in W. F. Bynum and Roy Porter (eds.), *William Hunter and the eighteenth-century medical world*, Cambridge University Press, 1985, pp. 153–76. For its relation to Scottish cultural life generally see Christopher Lawrence, 'The nervous system and society in the Scottish Enlightenment', in Barry Barnes and Steven Shapin (eds.), *Natural order: historical studies of scientific culture*, Beverly Hills, Sage Publications, 1979, pp. 19–40. For the suggestion that the great days were coming to an end in the 1790s see Christopher Lawrence, 'The Edinburgh medical school and the end of the "old thing", 1790–1830', *History of universities*, 1988, **7**: 259–86.

[44] The practice of medicine was a course of lectures and not a practical course.

[45] R. G. W. Anderson, *The Playfair collection and the teaching of chemistry at the University of Edinburgh, 1713–1858*, Edinburgh, Royal Scottish Museum, 1978, ch. 2.

[46] On the Edinburgh professors who were teaching in the 1790s see John D. Comrie, *History of Scottish medicine*, 2 vols., London, Wellcome Historical Medical Museum/Baillière, Tindall & Cox, 1932, vol. 2, pp. 628–31.

[47] For Edinburgh students and the courses they took, and an account of the extra mural school see

Edinburgh also had no formal overall course structure. Students simply matriculated (not all did that) and then attended whichever lectures they chose after paying the professor 3 guineas. They could also attend clinical lectures at the Royal Infirmary after having purchased a "ticket", a card bought from the Infirmary managers for a fee and giving the student the right to enter the Infirmary.[48] Students matriculating at Edinburgh did so in November when they signed the matriculation album in the University library. Woodforde signed his name in the 1791 album. He also signed the matriculation index and next to his name was a list of the courses he intended to take. This list was made by a clerk. He was listed as attending anatomy and surgery, chemistry, the practice of medicine, obstetrics and clinical medicine. In 1792–93 he again appears in the index enrolled for anatomy and surgery, obstetrics, medical theory (the Institutes of Medicine) and clinical medicine. His signature does not appear in the matriculation album. In 1793–94 he appears once more in the index but not in the album. The smudged entry reveals he enrolled for botany and another course, possibly the practice of physic, but the class list does not confirm this. Class lists were the professor's personal record of students enrolled. According to the class lists, Woodforde attended the practice of medicine in 1791–92 only. The class lists for clinical medicine confirm he attended in 1791–92 and 1792–93 but not in 1793–94. No other class lists for this period survive.[49]

By March 1792, after he had been in Edinburgh six months, Woodforde had decided to stay until September (letter **22**). Although there were no formal university lectures in the summer, there were extra-mural lectures and the infirmary could be visited. By June 1792 Woodforde was expressing a dislike of surgery and had decided to practise solely as an apothecary. He resolved to spend a second year in Edinburgh. Fothergill encouraged him to do whatever he wished but suggested that if he spent a second year at the University he might consider becoming an MD (letter **24**). In fact, unknown to Fothergill, in 1783 the regulations had been changed, stipulating that candidates for the Edinburgh MD degree must have spent three years at a university, one of which should have been passed at Edinburgh.[50] Woodforde meanwhile was undecided about which career to follow. By December 1792 he had chosen (letter **27**) to graduate. On 10 November 1792, a year after his arrival, Woodforde became a member of the RMS. The RMS began formally in 1737 and received a Royal Charter in 1779. Organised and run by medical students, it was exclusive and widely recognised as having an important educational function. It was also the seat of fierce controversy, as when it was split in the 1780s over the so-called Brunonian doctrine, named after the Edinburgh-trained physician John Brown.[51] Some time in 1793 Woodforde presented to the Society a paper entitled 'Asphyxia submersorum', which was a discussion of cases of drowning with commentaries. This was the basis of

---

Lisa Rosner, *Medical education in the age of improvement: Edinburgh students and apprentices 1760–1826*, Edinburgh University Press, 1991.

48 A. Logan Turner, *Story of a great hospital: the Royal Infirmary of Edinburgh*, Edinburgh, Oliver and Boyd, 1937, ch. 9. On teaching in the Infirmary see Guenter B. Risse, *Hospital life in Enlightenment Scotland: care and teaching at the Royal Infirmary of Edinburgh*, Cambridge University Press, 1986.

49 Edinburgh University Library: Medical Matriculation Index volume 2, 1791–95; Da 35, class lists, practice of medicine 1791–92, 1792–93, 1793–94; Da 35, clinical medicine class lists, 1791–92, 1792–93, 1793–94. In all of these entries Woodforde's name is spelt without an "e".

50 Rosner, op. cit., note 47 above, p. 63.

51 On the RMS see ibid, ch. 7. On the Brunonian controversy see Michael Barfoot, 'Brunonianism under

Woodforde's MD thesis and he was using the RMS to rehearse for his viva. At some point in the academic year 1793–94 he presented a dissertation, 'Why are the animal functions abolished in apoplexy while those of the vital and natural remain?'[52] In February 1793 Fothergill, having learned from Woodforde of the three years university attendance required for graduation, suggested he proceed to Leyden and graduate there (letters **28, 29, 30**). Prior to the rise of Edinburgh, Leyden was undoubtedly the premier European medical school. Hermann Boerhaave, who died in 1738, taught there and was one of the most admired and distinguished physicians of the century.[53] It was quite common in the eighteenth century to graduate at a university without having attended it. Rheims, like Leyden, was another popular choice for graduation. Fothergill offered Woodforde an interest-free loan of £10 to assist him in extra study. By June 1793 Fothergill had learned that Woodforde would stay in Edinburgh another year. Much of the correspondence in Woodforde's last academic year was taken up with the issue of his thesis and the oral examination, both of which would have to be in Latin and were necessary for graduation. By the summer of 1794 he had been examined and was an MD, his dissertation being dedicated to Fothergill and the founder of the Royal Humane Society, William Hawes (letter **36**). In September Woodforde was back in the West Country (letters **37** and **38**). Much of the correspondence from here on was devoted to attempts by Fothergill to introduce Woodforde to established local practitioners or to getting him an appointment of some sort, such as at a hospital (letters **37, 41, 49**). The correspondents, now on a more equal footing, continued to exchange books, pamphlets and, increasingly, journals. They also discussed medical cases. By May 1796 Woodforde was in practice in Castle Cary, Somerset (letter **50**). In 1799, the year of his mother's death, he moved to Crewkerne, also in Somerset (letter **67**). This latter caused Fothergill some surprise, since he considered Woodforde might have some difficulty attracting patients.

There is slightly less correspondence after 1799 although it seems certain letters have been either lost or were simply not transcribed. In 1802 Woodforde's wife announced she was expecting a baby (letter **78**) which was born in October (letter **80**). In 1803 Fothergill fell sick with "epidemic catarrh" (letter **81**), an illness from which he felt his recovery was unduly slow. His state of ill-health encouraged him in his decision to leave for Philadelphia (letter **82**). Fothergill's last letter before departing was written in August 1803. There are five long letters from America during the period 1809–12, although correspondence from this period is obviously missing. At this time Woodforde was contemplating translating Thomas Sydenham. Fothergill meanwhile was expressing satisfaction with his life of ease (letter **85**). By 1810 Woodforde had 5 children (letter **87**) and was considering a translation of Morgagni (or perhaps just to read it in the original) (letter **88**). The correspondence closes with two letters from London in 1813,

---

the bed; an alternative to university medicine in Edinburgh in the 1780s', in W. F. Bynum and Roy Porter (eds.), *Brunonianism in Britain and Europe*, London, *Medical History* Supplement No. 8, London, Wellcome Institute for the History of Medicine, 1988, pp. 22–45.

[52] Royal Medical Society, Edinburgh. 'Asphyxia submersorum', in volume 30 of Cases with Commentaries, commencing January 1793, p. 259. Woodforde's paper was question 3, suggesting it was presented in 1793. 'Animal functions', dissertations, 1792–1794, volume 29, pp. 431–43. Woodforde's paper was last in the volume, suggesting it was 1794.

[53] E. Ashworth Underwood, *Boerhaave's men at Leyden and after*, Edinburgh University Press, 1977.

on the second of which Woodforde wrote "the last from my dear valuable and ever to be revered friend and patron" (letter **91**).

Woodforde's health was a recurrent source of concern to Fothergill and it is frequently discussed in the letters. In early 1790 letter **4** gave the first indication of Woodforde's sickly disposition, which was to manifest itself in overt illness on several occasions. This illness had been overcome by April (letter **5**). In October 1792 Fothergill was concerned about Woodforde's indisposition of the "hypochondriacal kind" (letter **25**). Early in 1794 Woodforde fell ill again (letter **34**) and in 1802 he had a fever and pulmonary haemorrhage (letter **77**). In spite of the correspondence being full of local detail, it is surprising how little reference there is to other distinguished Bath physicians. Caleb Hillier Parry for example, who lived and practised in Bath during the whole time Fothergill was there, got no mention. John Haygarth who retired to Bath in 1798 is mentioned only once and not in any personal manner (letter **67**).

A Note on the Letterbook and our Transcription

Although the letters in the letterbook are clearly from Anthony Fothergill to James Woodforde, they are not originals but transcriptions. This is obvious since many letters begin on the page on which others end. The whereabouts of the originals is unknown. We have also been unable to trace Woodforde's letters to Fothergill. Fothergill's papers were acquired by John Coakley Lettsom but then all record of them disappears. The letterbook has no provenance beyond the fact that it was acquired by Whitfield Bell Jr. in 1972 for the American Philosophical Society from a London manuscripts and autograph dealer. The transcriptions are deeply puzzling. At one point (letter **60**) Woodforde declared his intention to transcribe Fothergill's letters. If he did so these transcriptions are not they. These seem to have been made by someone relatively illiterate and unacquainted with the details of the Woodforde family's life. It seems impossible that they were made by any of Woodforde's sons unless it was in their dotage. The letters are numbered and very often have a date; however, the dates are not always in sequence and often do not correspond to the actual calendar (for example, letter **67**, November 9 was not a Saturday in 1798). This, coupled with various internal material contradictions, has led us to rearrange and renumber the letters for a reading closer to what we think was the original sequence. Accordingly, the letterbook numbering in its original form (as in N° 1, N° 2 etc.) has been retained for information and a new sequential numbering added in bold. We have added two tables correlating the two sets of numbers. For the most part we feel we have recovered the original sequence although some letters defy placement and may well not be part of the Fothergill-Woodforde correspondence (notably letter **84**). We have also indicated what we consider more accurate dating by using square brackets.

We originally intended to publish an exact transcription of the letterbook. However it became increasingly apparent to us that the originals themselves must have differed in many minor ways from the letterbook version. First the transcriber was not familiar with the medical world in which Woodforde and Fothergill lived. Medical terms and the names of famous medical men (especially foreigners) are frequently and often badly misspelt and, what is more, misspelt in different ways. Even allowing for eighteenth-century idiosyncratic spelling, Anthony Fothergill was far too cultivated a physician to have written so sloppily.

Second, the transcriber almost certainly had no Latin. Practically every Latin tag contains an error, sometimes quite gross. Fothergill obviously prided himself on his Latin, as the letters indicate, and he encouraged the young Woodforde to perfect himself in the language. That the transcriber seems to have had no intimate knowledge of the Woodforde family is evidenced in numerous places, notably in letter **28** where James is referred to as John. There are many other puzzles, not least that the transcriber was not only unacquainted with the family but seemingly forgot what had already been transcribed. In letters **63–66** in 1798, Fothergill expressed concern for Woodforde's sick mother, who did indeed die shortly afterwards (letter **67**). In letter **89**, written from Philadelphia in 1812, Fothergill enquired after Woodforde's mother. Possibly Fothergill was becoming very forgetful. Possibly he was enquiring about Woodforde's mother-in-law. Possibly it was a thoughtless transcription of brother. This along with countless other oddities has led us to publish the letters in what we consider is a form closer to the originals.

We have made no major alterations, but we have modified some spellings (leaving certain inconsistencies), corrected the Latin, adjusted the punctuation and in a few places altered the grammar. We have omitted nothing. There are ninety numbered letters in all. A consultation letter, also in the letterbook, from the Edinburgh surgeon James Russell, presumably, but not certainly, to Woodforde, is not numbered but has been included in the appropriate place by date (letter **48**).[54] In sum, however, there are very many minor alterations and to have indicated them all would have cluttered the text to an extent that would have made easy, let alone pleasurable, reading impossible. We have tried to identify all people and books mentioned in the letters. All appearances are noted in the index but biographical information or bibliographical details are recorded on the first occasion only, unless it seemed particularly pertinent to repeat them. People mentioned who are unknown to us have not been footnoted. Our title is the injunction Fothergill repeats more than once to his protégé (letters **15, 20, 31**).

Bound in with the letterbook and possibly in a different hand and newly paginated is another document (item **92**). It is the deposition of a person, presumably Woodforde, to the Royal Commission appointed to enquire into the state of the jail at Ilchester, Somerset, in 1820. We have included it, without annotation or correction, for the sake of completeness.

[54] This letter is not numbered in the original but appears between letters no. 88 and no. 89, starting on the page on which no. 88 finishes and ending on the page on which no. 89 starts. This suggests it was in this place in the original letters since the transcriber seems to have transcribed the letters in the order he or she found them. We have given it a number of 88a (**48**) to situate it in the letterbook sequence.

The Letters

N° 1 **1**

Bath August 26 1789

Before me, kind sir, is your very obliging letter in which your politeness has induced you to overrate my abilities, and to apply to me encomiums which justly belong to my late illustrious and ever to be revered namesake,[1] whose character you wish to emulate—and a better model I am certain you could not have chosen in the whole catalogue of medical worthies.

Tho' much pressed for time with a large packet of letters and pending engagements before me, yet I cannot defer testifying my warmest approbation of that generous zeal and enthusiasm which you express for medical science. From this I dare, almost, venture to prognosticate your future excellence, and that you will probably one day prove an ornament to the profession you have chosen.

If any hint of mine towards regulating the objects of your studies can prove conducive to your success, or expedite your progress, be assured, it will afford me much pleasure.

If you will lay before me a list of your books, marking those you have read, and can determine at present whether you intend to qualify yourself for a physician, surgeon or apothecary, I will communicate such observations as may occur to me on the subject.

If you have had a good classical education, this will be a good foundation for any of the three branches and greatly facilitate your future studies. If you mean to be a physician, and your income will permit, I should advise you to have a very complete education on the most liberal plan and to complete it by foreign travel, attending the most eminent professors at Leyden and Paris, after you have graduated at Edinburgh. Meanwhile I must caution you against indiscriminate reading which, as you justly observe, bewilders young students and leads to confusion. Nor is this all; erroneous ideas are often thus imbibed at an early period, and it requires no small trouble and mortification afterwards to "unlearn what has been learnt amiss."

Whatever may be your destination, a proper plan and method of study is indispensably necessary, hence the great advantage of a regular education over the vague and undigested notions obtained from desultory reading. With comp^{ts} to Messrs Palmer and Silvester.[2] I am Sir, yours very sincerely. A. Fothergill

[1] John Fothergill (1712–1780), MD, FRS, Quaker, London practitioner, philanthropist and botanist.
[2] William Palmer (1710–1792) and Joseph Sylvester (1730–1798), apothecary-surgeons of Trowbridge, Wiltshire. James Woodford (no e) was apprenticed to them 11 May 1786. See P. J. and R. V. Wallis, *Eighteenth century medics*, Newcastle upon Tyne, Project for Historical Biobibliography, 1988, p. 449.

N° 2 **2**

Bath 3rd September 1789

Kind Sir,

As you place so much confidence in my opinion, I will endeavour as far as my time will

allow, to answer the most material passages in your last obliging letter relative to the course of your studies.

Considering you as the youngest of seven children and the disadvantages under which you have laboured in being deprived of the opportunity of acquiring a proper classical education, I cannot but admire the progress you have already made by mere dint of genius and unwearied application. I am pleased to find so very few slips of the pen in your letters, making allowance for these (and great allowance ought certainly to be made), you express yourself, on the whole, with much force, and propriety

> "Ubi plurima nitent
> Non ego paucis offendar maculis."[1]

and for your consolation I must further add that I have known surgeons and apothecaries of considerable note express themselves with much less correctness and perspicuity. But such are by no means patterns for you who will, I dare say, study to avoid their inaccuracies and strive to imitate the correctness and precision of D[r] J. Fothergill and other excellent authors. Tho' it may not be easy, or even necessary to obtain their elegance of style and composition, yet grammatical accuracy seems indispensable. If you read over once or twice with attention Lowth's English Grammar[2] you will find your labour not ill bestowed; and as a tolerable knowledge of Latin is highly requisite and perhaps, I may add, the rudiments of the Greek tongue, without which it is almost impossible to understand a variety of anatomical, medical and botanical terms immediately derived from these languages, you will do well to set apart some portion of your time in acquiring at least the elements. You may think this retrograde plan rather mortifying but, be assured, it will be more agreeable and satisfactory in the end, than to leave it to begin at a more advanced period of life. After the English grammar it will be right to reperuse the Latin one and accompany it with some easy school book, as Erasmus, Cornelius Nepos, Terence and others, and to try your proficiency by translating Latin into English, and vice versa. This with your other indispensable avocations will not leave much time for promiscuous reading and the less perhaps the better, tho' I am far from thinking that the labour you have already bestowed in this way is wholly thrown away, only misplaced. Whoever means to acquire useful medical knowledge must be content to learn it methodically and begin with languages, the A.B.C. of this, and every other science. A good foundation thus laid, the superstructure will follow in good order. As your destination is surgery, pharmacy and perhaps midwifery, your next object of attention ought to be anatomy beginning with osteology, the basis of anatomy. The best book in this subject is Monro's Osteology[3] which should be carefully compared with the different parts of the skeleton beginning with the cranium. After this treatise on the muscles with Albinus's tables,[4] next Winslow.[5] Further you cannot proceed with advantage till you attend a regular course of anatomy, or even two, which with dissection will complete your inquiries on that important branch of study. It will be best to avoid all miscellaneous reading for the present, till you are well grounded in the elements of medicine, a course of natural philosophy would be an excellent introduction. Would your time allow of it, I should recommend a previous perusal of 'sGravesande's,[6] Nicholson's,[7] or Enfield's[8] experimental philosophy. This by unfolding general principles enlarges the ideas, and is intimately connected with every branch of medicine. Wishing you success in all your undertakings, I remain, Sir, yours very sincerely

A. Fothergill

[1] "Where most things are brilliant, I shall not be worried by a few blemishes", Horace, *Art of poetry*, 351–2.

[2] One of the many editions of Robert Lowth (1710–1787), bishop of London, *A short introduction to English grammar; with critical notes*, London, A. Millar and R. & J. Dodsley, 1762. New editions published in 1764, 1769, 1771, 1775, 1781, 1783, 1786 and 1787.

[3] One of the editions of Alexander Monro, *primus* (1697–1767), *The anatomy of the humane bones*, Edinburgh, T. Ruddiman for W. Munro, 1726. Many subsequent editions. See K. F. Russell, *British anatomy, 1525–1800*, 2nd ed., Winchester, St. Paul's Bibliographies, 1987.

[4] Bernhard Siegfried Albinus (1697–1770), *Tables of the skeleton and muscles of the human body. . . . Translated from the Latin*, London, H. Woodfall, for J. & P. Knapton, 1749. Another edition, Edinburgh, 1777–8.

[5] Jacques Bénigne Winslow (1669–1760), *An anatomical exposition of the structure of the human body . . . Translated . . . by G. Douglas*, 2 vols., London, Printed for N. Prevost, 1723. "The fifth edition", London, 1776. See Russell, this letter, note 3.

[6] Presumably one of the many editions of Willem Jakob Storm van 'sGravesande (1688–1742), *Mathematical elements of natural philosophy, confirmed by experiments, or, an introduction to Sir Isaac Newton's philosophy, written in Latin by William James 'sGravesande . . . Translated into English by J. T. Desaguliers*, 2 vols., London, J. Senex & W. Taylor, 1720. Sixth edition, 1747.

[7] William Nicholson (1753–1815), *An introduction to natural philosophy*, 2 vols., London, n.p., 1782. Second edition, London, J. Johnson, 1787.

[8] William Enfield (1741–1797), *Institutes of natural philosophy, theoretical and experimental*, London, J. Johnson, 1785.

N° 3 **3**

Bath October 18th 1789

Dear Sir,

I was favoured with your kind letter of the 12th and am pleased to find that you can so readily reconcile yourself to the humiliating task of refreshing your memory concerning the elements of the English and Latin tongues. But although this at first view may appear a retrograde method of study, be assured you will find it hereafter very beneficial, and as you proceed will, I make no doubt, be more and more convinced of its propriety. For without solid foundation, no permanent superstructure can ever be raised. Therefore I think it will be very proper to peruse Lowth once more with <u>attention</u> and to try other English books and your own letters by his rules. After you have done this go through the Latin grammar leisurely, making yourself master of the rules by translating and retranslating as I mentioned before. Cornelius Nepos or Erasmus may assist you in these exercises, Rowning's philosophy[1] tho' deficient as to aer[l] fluids yet may do very well to give you the elements of natural philosophy on which you may also consult Pemberton[2] or M^claurin[3] on the Newtonian philosophy or even Martin.[4] But be not in too great haste as to the particular qualities of bodies. This is the business of chemistry, the elements of which must be regularly studied before you can profit by reading Priestley[5] or other writers on the abstruse parts of chemical science. Be content to learn the outlines and elements before you wade into the depths of philosophy and be careful as you proceed to <u>digest</u> the principles so as to fix them <u>in your memory</u> for on these the <u>whole system depends</u>. If you make yourself master of these <u>you</u> will then be well prepared to attend <u>lectures</u> in the different branches, and fully to comprehend the rationale of the experiments brought by the professor to illustrate each proposition. As natural philosophy unfolds the general properties of bodies, so chemistry explains the particular properties of bodies, and each mutually illustrates the other, and the method requires that we begin with the generals and gradually descend to particulars. Medicine embraces all the sciences and presupposes a general knowledge of each.

Hence the time, labour, and expense necessary to acquire a complete medical education!! "Ubi desinit philosophus, incipit medicus."[6]

At some leisure time it may not be improper to read Dr Gregory's Duties and Offices of a Physician,[7] notwithstanding your destination for surgery, because many of his excellent precepts apply equally to both physic and surgery. Tho' I applaud your ardour and enthusiasm for science yet let me give you one caution. Let not your zeal for study break in upon your hours of rest and necessary bodily exercise. For knowledge, however desirable, is too dearly purchased at the expense of health. This is not meant to damp your ardour, but to regulate it by the bounds of prudence. With best wishes for your success I remain,

Dear Sir much yours

A. Fothergill

[1] Presumably one of the many editions of John Rowning (1701?–1771), *A compendious system of natural philosophy*, Cambridge University Press, 1734. Sixth edition, 1767. This work was superseded by William Nicholson's, *Introduction to natural philosophy* (letter **2**, note 7), as an elementary class-book.

[2] Presumably, Henry Pemberton (1694–1771), *A view of Sir Isaac Newton's philosophy*, London, S. Palmer, 1728.

[3] One of the editions of Colin Maclaurin (1698–1746), *An account of Sir Isaac Newton's philosophical discoveries*, London, P. Murdoch, 1748.

[4] Possibly one of the editions of Benjamin Martin (1705–82), *A course of lectures in natural and experimental philosophy, geography and astronomy: in which the properties, affections, and phaenomena of natural bodies . . . are exhibited and explain'd on the principles of the Newtonian philosophy*, Reading, J. Newbery & C. Micklewright, 1743; or, *Philosophia Britannica; or, a new . . . system of the Newtonian philosophy, astronomy and geography*, 2 vols., Reading, C. Micklewright & Co., 1747; or, *The young gentleman and lady's philosophy, in a continued survey of the works of nature and art; by way of a dialogue*, 2 vols., London, W. Owen [& the author], 1755–63.

[5] Joseph Priestley (1733–1804), LL.D. (Edinburgh 1762), FRS, theologian and chemist, and member of the Birmingham Lunar Society.

[6] "Where the philosopher stops, the physician begins". Although an ancient conception, this dictum was a Renaissance coining. There are many variants and its origins are obscure. See C. B. Schmitt, 'Aristotle among the physicians', in A. Wear, R. K. French and I. M. Lonie (eds.), *The medical renaissance of the sixteenth century*, Cambridge University Press, 1985, pp. 1–15.

[7] John Gregory (1724–1773) [Anon], *Observations on the duties and offices of a physician; and on the method of prosecuting enquiries in philosophy*, London, W. Strahan & T. Cadell, 1770. This was an unauthorized edition, published from notes taken at Gregory's lectures in Edinburgh. Gregory then published an edition under his own name, *Lectures on the duties and qualifications of a physician, a new edition . . . enlarged*, London, W. Strahan & T. Cadell, 1772.

N° 5 **4**

Bath Janry 13th 1790

Before me, kind sir, is your very obliging letter, which a variety of professional and other letters have obliged me to postpone till now. It is with pleasure I observe a very visible improvement in your style and orthography which strongly evinces that you have already availed yourself of the authors recommended to your perusal, and have profited not a little by their instructions. In your last I only observe two little slips of the pen which, for your satisfaction, I shall point out: "fell a victim to them very frequent" instead of "those very frequent", again "nervous complaints which seems" instead of "seem".

Remember a noun of the plural number requires a verb of the plural number and vice versa. Please to go thro' Lowth once more and examine yourself on each rule and example. But first of all let me entreat you to take more care of your health, and to set apart at least 1 hour for bodily exercise; and not to suffer study to encroach on this, or the hours of rest. As your habit is constitutionally delicate this precaution will be the more necessary. If you drive off natural sleep by intense application, a habit of watching will certainly ensue. Resolve therefore to make study rather a pleasing amusement than a severe labour.

Close the book an hour before bedtime and banish all concern about it till the morning following, and if the watching still continues take before you go to rest of Syrupi Papaveris Albi 3 to 4 drachms[1] and if you use exercise in the open air every day, you'll soon find your natural rest will be restored without any opiate.—"In which engaged in"—delete the last "in", which is tautology. You may spare the expense of buying the rules of health falsely attributed to D^r^ J[ohn]F[othergill].[2] He assured me the work was spurious, and felt himself so much hurt by the imputation of such a catch-penny performance that he advertised his total [word missing] of the shameless author. In the next number of the Literary Magazine will appear a portrait of this excellent man whose conduct was so truly amiable that, as Shakespeare expresses it, "we scarcely shall see his like again."[3] From your account you have, I find, dipped deeper into anatomy than could reasonably be expected in so short a time, and by which you will find yourself well prepared for an anatomical course, and be able sometimes to anticipate the professor in his demonstrations. Suppose you take a little time to breathe before you engage in any fresh study, and at leisure times take a retrospect of what you have already read, and examine yourself as you go along not only in grammar but also anatomy. There was lately published a very useful book for the rudiments of anatomy and physiology called a Breviary of Anatomy in Form of Dialogue,[4] which is of all others the best plan of fixing in the mind the first principles. When you have carefully perused it, you may examine yourself by the book which perfectly agrees with what I have been recommending. I hear a good account of the work but have not seen it. The above, together with the Latin grammar and Latin exercises, will be more than sufficient to occupy your leisure hours (and these only can be properly spared from the duties of your profession for some time to come) even without natural philosophy of which 'sGravesande's Introduction to the Newtonian Philosophy is a short useful compendium of the first principles and not high priced. But beware of too many irons in the fire at once, and take care of your health, without which, science will but little avail you. I have barely room to add my best wishes for your prosperity and success. A. Fothergill.

P.S. After you are well grounded in your present studies (a work of much time and patience) it will be then time enough to proceed to practical authors in medicine, which properly come last of all and indeed cannot be well understood until principles are unfolded. When you are master of these, I may perhaps lend you the journals and commentaries. A.F.

[1] Syrup of white poppy, containing opium. Fothergill gives the quantities in the signs for Apothecary measures.

[2] The spuriously attributed, *Rules for the preservation of health*, London, J. Pridden, 1762, which went through several editions.

[3] Hamlet, of his father, "I shall not look upon his like again". *Hamlet*, I, 2, 188.

[4] Probably, *Anatomical dialogues; or, a breviary of anatomy . . .Chiefly compiled for the use of the young*

gentlemen in the Navy and Army. By a gentleman of the faculty, London, printed for G. Robinson, 1778; second edition, 1785.

N° 4 **5**

Bath April 1790

Dear Sir,

Before me is your last long and very obliging letter, which with many others I have been obliged, thro' extreme hurry, to postpone till now, and shall consider them in their order so far as my time will allow. But my kind correspondents must not expect adequate returns for their esteemed favours, but content themselves with receiving short answers.

In the first place, I am much pleased to hear so favorable an account of your health, and that your natural rest is returned, and with it your former alacrity of mind and body which enables you to prosecute your studies with pleasure and success. Your duty and affection for your mother affords me peculiar satisfaction, in which, I hope, you will ever continue to imitate the amiable Atticus, as this was perhaps one of the most engaging traits in the character of that most accomplished Roman. I hope your dear mother is perfectly recovered and that you will not forget in your next letter to return my best acknowledgements for her kind expressions of gratitude.

Your motive for beginning early with practical writers, contrary to the rules of right order, was a venial, nay, an amiable fault, and carries with it more than an apology. It was making a virtue of necessity which could not be properly resisted. There can be no fear of your acquiring a competent knowledge of Latin by setting apart an hour every day for that purpose. The professors at Edinburgh formerly lectured in Latin chiefly, now all in English. For the Scotch pronunciation of Latin is uncouth to an English ear. But could wish you to take a few instructions on your setting out, from some eminent grammarian as to the improved methods of obtaining the rudiments with ease and expedition, otherwise some time may be lost. Perhaps the Reverend Mr Batchelor (a worthy, which is in your favour, teacher at Freshford)[1] might condescend to give you the outlines much better than I can pretend to do, as he doubtless has considered the different methods and can point out the best.

You must not at present attempt minutiæ of anatomy; gain but a tolerable knowledge of the principal parts and leave the rest till you can see them demonstrated in a course of lectures.

Dr Cleghorn's[2] death which happened lately in Ireland is a real loss to science. I have read his excellent observations on the diseases of Minorca[3] but never saw his anatomical dialogues,[4] and may perhaps accept your kind offer when leisure shall permit.

If you can spare one hour for Latin, one for anatomy, and another for natural philosy daily, it will, with your necessary business, occupy the chief part of your time, and I hope very usefully. Besides 'sGravesande there is Ferguson's Introduction,[5] Martin's Dialogues for Young Gentlemen in Philosophy, later works, and perhaps less dry, but I've not seen them. Also Nicholson's, still later, and well spoken of. The first was the textbook used at Edinburgh by professor Ferguson,[6] since professor of moral philosophy. Euclid's Elements ought properly to precede every other, being the basis of the science of mathematical knowledge but it wou'd take up too much time and require a master often at your elbow. In short, you may gain a tolerable knowledge of the subject without it, which is all you can expect at present, or is indeed essential. As to your important question concerning Edinburgh, as you have the concurrence of your friends, I cannot hesitate in warmly recommending so desirable a scheme. The lectures there only commence on the 29th of October and the first week is taken up with the history of the different branches of physic, which is, however entertaining, if not essential. Whatever may be your future destination, your motives are laudable, and your reasoning concerning the weighty trust that daily devolves on apothecaries, perfectly just. When I left Edinburgh in 1764 young gentlemen boarded and lodged from 16^{s} to 1 G per week which saved much trouble and was nearly as cheap as finding provisions oneself. To each of the professors about 3 Guineas a course, Infirmary 3 Guin^{s}, clinical lectures 2 G^{s}, botany 2 G^{s}. Perhaps board is now higher from the advanced rates of provisions but still doubtless cheaper than London. A new College is now erecting[7] and this may add something, also 1 G. to the Lib^{y} and admission into the Medical Society, of which if you can get admitted soon, it will be a great acquisition. But more of this before you start. In your long letter I observe but a single slip and that a slight one "acquiesce to it", pro "in" it. I cannot conclude without expressing my warmest satisfaction in observing that your improvement keeps pace with your diligence. "Nil tam difficile est quod non solertia vincat."[8] That your health may permit you to proceed in your career with alacrity is the sincere wish of, Dr Sir, yours

A. Fothergill

[1] Reverend Batchelor of Freshford, Somerset. A number of candidates suggest themselves, notably Joseph Batchelor (matriculated Pembroke College, Oxford, 1773) or his brother William (BA Oxon 1780), sons of William, clerk, of Trowbridge, Wiltshire, or John Batchelor (matriculated St Edmund Hall, Oxford, 1783) (possibly another brother) son of William, clerk, of Tellisford, Somerset. See J. A. Venn, *Alumni Cantabrigienses*, Part II, of 4 vols., Cambridge University Press, 1940–51, vol. 1 p. 181, and Joseph Foster, *Alumni Oxoniensis*, Series 2, 2 vols., Nendeln/Liechtenstein, Klause Reprint Limited, 1968, vol. 1, p. 73.

[2] George Cleghorn (1716–1789), MD (Edinburgh 1779), settled in Dublin in 1751, later became professor of anatomy in the university.

[3] Idem, *Observations on the epidemical diseases in Minorca. From the year 1744 to 1749. To which is prefixed, a short account of the climate, productions, inhabitants, and endemial distempers of that island*, London, D.Wilson, 1751. Four editions were published in Cleghorn's lifetime.

[4] Unclear reference, perhaps, George Cleghorn, *Index of an annual course of lectures*, Dublin, printed by William Sleater, printer to the University, 1756; another edition, 1757.

[5] James Ferguson (1710–1776), *Lectures on select subjects in mechanics, hydrostatics, pneumatics, and optics*, London, A. Millar, 1760; seventh edition, 1790; or *An introduction to electricity*, London, W. Strahan & T. Cadell, 1770; or, *The young gentleman and lady's astronomy. Familiarly explained in ten dialogues*, London, A. Millar & T. Cadell, 1768, all later English editions (except 1815) entitled *An easy introduction to astronomy, for young gentlemen and ladies*; second edition, 1769.

[6] Adam Ferguson (1723–1816), LL.D., appointed professor of natural philosophy in the university of Edinburgh in 1759, and appointed professor of moral philosophy in 1764.

[7] New university buildings had been approved by the Senate in 1768. The cost was to be raised by subscription. The plan failed for financial reasons. In 1789 the town council again tried to raise money for new buildings for which the architect Robert Adam had already circulated designs. Demolition and rebuilding began in early 1790 as Fothergill's letter records. Financial problems and differences between Adam and the builders dogged the project. Adam died in 1792. Early in 1794 the work came to a halt, only a small number of buildings being completed. Others were left quite unfinished. See A. J. Youngson, *The making of classical Edinburgh*, 1750–1840, Edinburgh University Press, 1966, pp. 123–32.

[8] "There is no difficulty so great that ingenuity does not overcome it". Proverb.

N° 7 **6**

Bath June 19th 1790

Dear Sir

During my absence in London on indispensable business your letter arrived, since which my numerous engagements have left me no time to answer it till this moment. I have, however, run over the principal parts of the second vol. you sent, and now return them with thanks. Both appear to me very useful compendiums, written in a easy, clear and agreeable manner, and every way worthy of the idea I had formed of them. The form of dialogue engages attention, assists the memory, and enables the reader to exercise his abilities in anticipating the answer. Such works are useful not only to those who are beginning the study, but also to those who have completed it, by recalling many things to mind which had been once learnt, but since wholly lost. Before you attend a course of lectures on natural philosophy and anatomy, it will be advisable to give the volumes a 2nd perusal, examining yourself as you proceed on the several questions.

Some few errors will occur, but the general tenor will be found incontrovertible. I have not seen Martin's other vol^{s} nor Nicholson's Phil^{y} but from the character I have heard of them I hope they will ans^{r} y^{r} expectation and supersede the necess^{y} of purchasing any more books on the subject. When you have carefully read these, you may begin Haller's Primae Lineae as physiol^{y} naturally succeeds anat^{y}, beautifully illustrating the functions of the animated machine, and explaining the several parts you have been contemplating in the dead subject If you have not Dr Cullen's Edit^{n} and notes on Haller's Primae Lineae[1] I can lend it you and also Haller's Prelections or Comment^{y} on his First Lines,[2] a large and important work, but in Latin, and therefore must be postponed till you have learnt the language. Towards which the books recommended by M^{r} B[atchelor?] seem extremely well adapted, now that you are master of Lowth's English Grammar which you'll find will facilitate your progress not a little. I attended Dr Blair's Belles Lettres[3] as a delightful relaxation for some severer studies, but this must be postponed. For the present, an hour sh^{d} be spent daily on the rudiments of Latin, another in tracing the blood vessels and afterwards the nerves, if you have any tolerable good plates. This will be a good preparative for a course of anat^{y} and the physiol^{y} will illustrate and impress it on your memory. If you have no anatomical plates I can lend you the 5th vol of the new Cyclopædia which contains the plates of ye whole work on all the sciences.[4] I meet with two or three little inaccuracies in y^{r} lett^{r}, but too slight to require animadversion.

"Non ego paucis offendar maculis" <u>Horace</u>[5]

Your remarks on the absurd variety of weights and measures are very just. This subject is now before both the British and French Parlim^{ts}, a subject in which all Europe is concerned and w^{h}, it is hoped, will be thoroughly discussed, and grievance removed. Y^{r} strictures on bell-metal mortars are also proper. As you express a wish to see my new tract; ye Poison of Lead and Copper, I have herewith sent you a copy, tho' it is not yet published.[6] You may look it over, and circulate it among y^{r} friends to guard them against an evil of which few except the faculty are suffic^{y} aware. Nor are these at all times so attentive as might be wished, or indeed expected. This tract with a copy of Dr Hawes's address,[7] and my Hints on Animation are much at y^{r} service.[8] But I must once more caution you not to have "too many irons in the fire"—nor suffer even ye best practical or miscell^{s} writers to interfere with y^{r} preliminary studies. First make yourself master of those, and these will afterwards follow in due course.

My respects to y^{r} mother, and believe me, Dr Sir
much y^{rs} A. Fothergill

P.S. You have already read my 2nd ed^{n} on Cheltenham Waters.[9]

[1] William Cullen (1710–1790), professor of the practice of physic in the university of Edinburgh, *First lines of physiology. Translated from the correct Latin edition printed under the inspection of William Cullen*, Edinburgh, C. Elliot, 1779.

[2] Cullen's English edition was a complete translation of Albrecht von Haller (1708–1777), *Primae lineae physiologiae in usum praelectionum academicarum*, 3rd ed., Edinburgh, G. Drummond & Kincaid & Bell, 1767 (first edition, 1747). Fothergill's "commentary" was probably Haller's *Elementa physiologiae corporis humani*, 8 vols., Lausanne, M. M. Bousquet, S. d'Arnay, F. Grasset, Leyden, C. Haak, 1757–66.

[3] Hugh Blair (1718–1800), D.D., since 1762 Regius professor of rhetoric and belles lettres in the university of Edinburgh.

[4] Presumably, *Cyclopædia: or, an universal dictionary of arts and sciences . . . With the supplement and modern improvements, incorporated in one alphabet, by A. Rees*, 5 vols., London, W. Strahan & T. Cadell, 1778–88.

[5] "I shall not be worried by a few blemishes". Horace, *Art of poetry*, 351–2. See also letter **2**.

[6] Anthony Fothergill, *Cautions to the heads of families in three essays: (I.) On cyder-wine . . . (II.) On the poison of lead . . .(III.) On the poison of copper . . .* Bath, R. Cruttwell, 1790.

[7] William Hawes (1736–1808), MD, founder of the Royal Humane Society and physician to the London Dispensary. Presumably, one of several possible addresses: (1) *An address on premature death and premature interment*, 1777; (2) *An address to the public on the dangerous custom of laying out persons as soon as respiration ceases, with a reply by W. Renwick, and observations on that reply*, 1778; (3) *An address to the legislature on the importance of a Humane Society*, 1781; or (4) *An address to the King and Parliament of Great Britain on the important subject of preserving the lives of its inhabitants*, 1782; third edition, *to which are now added observations on the general bills of mortality*, 1783.

[8] Anthony Fothergill, *Hints for improving the art of restoring suspended animation*, London, 1782, first appeared subjoined to Hawes's address of that year, ibid.

[9] Idem, *A new experimental inquiry into the nature and qualities of the Cheltenham water*, 2nd ed., Bath, R. Cruttwell, 1788 (first edition, 1785).

N° 6 **7**

Bath July 5th 1790

Dear Sir,

About a week ago I returned your books by Mr Batchelor Junr accompanied with others, and a letter in answer to your last which you will find on your return, together with this, in which I have barely time to acknowledge your kind mother's very obliging, tho' totally unexpected present. But remember my wish to assist you in a method of study was never meant to become burthensome to her, my sole object was to direct your inquiries and expedite your improvement without any return on your part except now and then a letter to afford me an opportunity to judge concerning your progress. However as nothing short of this will, I see, satisfy grateful and susceptible minds, I accept the kind present with due acknowledgements. When you have perused Nicholson's Philosophy with care, you may send it, when opportunity offers, with the sequel of Martin's Philosophy and then I will acquaint you more how far these books answer, in my idea, the encomiums I have heard concerning them. But before you purchase any other books, I should wish to know whether they are to be found in my collection, that I may, if possible, spare you unnecessary expense on that head.

The unavoidable expense of a tolerably complete education, you will find sufficiently great. Therefore we must consider how every unnecessary expense may be properly avoided.

Your reflection of the importance of your time at this juncture, in order to insure a valuable reversion in future, is pointedly just, and merits remembrance in the prosecution of your studies. When you arrive at Edinburgh you will meet with many dissipated sons of fortune who will strive to throw every serious and laudable pursuit into ridicule and render you as ignorant and profligate as themselves.

I have already answered your question on Blair's Rhetoric.[1] The rudiments of Latin and anatomy are more than sufficient to employ your leisure hours at present. If you are impatient to run over my little tracts, they are short, and will not lose you much time, tho' I cannot tell how you can fully comprehend them at present.[2] When you have attended a course of chemistry you will then be prepared to give them a second perusal. I observe what you say concerning Mr Long and am sensible of your goodwill, but I fear Mr Long has not resolution to go thro' a course of medicine necessary to his complete recovery. I wish for his own sake, that he may, with best wishes to your affectionate mother. I am Dr Sir yours assuredly. A. Fothergill.

N.B. you say my mother and self sends &c. instead of send, a noun of the plural with a verb of the singular—see Lowth's Grammar.

[1] Hugh Blair, *Lectures on rhetoric and belles lettres*, 2 vols., London, W. Strahan & T. Cadell, 1783; second edition, 1785; third, 1787; fourth, 1790; or, *Essays on rhetoric: abridged chiefly from Dr. Blair's lectures on that science*, London, J. Murray, 1785; second edition, 1785; third, 1787.

[2] See letter **6**, notes 6, 7, 8 and 9.

Nº 8 **8**

Bath August 18th 1790

Dear Sir

I have barely time to acknowledge the favour of your very obliging letter accompd by Martin and Nicholson both which shall be glanced over as opporty may offer, and returned safely. I observe with pleasure your progress in yr studies and see nothing to correct in your letters, tho' very long, except in certain passages where you continue as usual greatly to overrate the supposed merit and abilities of yr instructor who daily finds sufficient reason to think very humbly of both, and to lament that his progress in science has been so very disproportionate to his years and opportunities of improvement. Herewith you'll receive Haller's Physioly by Cullen 2 vols in 1, with Wrisberg's notes,[1] which must be perused with attention, looking back to the references. It contains the 1st elemts of the science in a condensed form and is a work of immense labour and must have cost long and laborious reading as you'll find when you come afterwards to read Haller's large work in 8 vol. 4to;[2] an excellent commentary on these first lines. But the Latin is crabbed and obscure and will require further grammatical knowledge preparatory to its being read with facility, for we have no English translation. I am glad friend Stonhouse, who was my very eminent predecessor at North^{n}, has presented you with C. Nepos and that his son Timothy has written you a polite letter.[3] When you have finished 'sGraves^{de} and Rowning you may be supposed to have laid a good foundation in the rudiments of exper^{l} philosophy which a single course of lectures, when you can spare time, will complete. On looking over the plates of the Cyclopædia, I find all the anatomical figures crowded into one plate and so miserably deficient that they wou'd rather lead you into error, or wou'd have sent the volume. Nor have I any on the nerves or blood vessels that I can recommend. Haller's will cost 5 G^{s} merely for the blood vessels; you'll see it and Meckel[?][4] at Edin^{r} in the Lib^{y} and what is better, the real subject accurately dissected and demonstrated. As to the lymphat^{s}, when you have gone thro' Haller's Elem^{s} I can lend you Hewson's 3 vol^{s};[5] an excellent work, but I have not Cruikshank's[6] or Sheldon.[7] I think the application of spirits with a suitable bandage likely to answer in checking superfluous osseous matter, as you rightly conjecture. But Bell in his Surgery[8] may perhaps suggest more approved means. The softness of bones arises from a defect of ossification and cannot be remedied but by invigorating the habit and that, I fear, but in a very imperfect degree.

In digestion the gastric juice possesses a real solvent power and perhaps approaches nearer to an universal menstruum than any boasted of by the chemists, but whether a peculiar fermentation may not be also requisite to assimilate the various aliments into one homogeneous chyle and complete the process of digestion, I am not without some doubts. It yet remains sub judice whether the principle of irritability is wholly independent of the nerves as Haller asserts from direct exper^{ts}.[9] But exper^{ts} of this nature are liable to fallacy, and I think this principle is materially if not wholly connected with nervous energy, and that this energy depends on a very subtile fluid, the nature of which is wholly unknown.[10] Omit Bell's anatomical plates[11] till we hear more of their merit. The Scotch plates are generally very coarse and slovenly executed as appears from some specimens I saw some time ago, Monro on the nerves and fishes &c &c.[12] If I should hear of any plates that may assist you I will let you know. You may take time with Moore[13] and Haller and proceed with your present important course, in w^{h} I wish you all imaginable success and am, Dear Sir, much yours

A. Fothergill

[1] Albrecht von Haller, *First lines of physiology translated from the correct Latin edition. Printed under the inspection of William Cullen, and compared with the edition published by H. A. Wrisberg*, 2 vols in 1 vol., Edinburgh, Elliot, 1786. The edition of Heinrich August Wrisberg (1739–1808) was *Primae lineae physiologiae auctae ab H. A. Wrisberg*, Göttingen, 1780.

[2] See letter **6**, note 2.

[3] Sir James Stonhouse (1716–1795), baronet, physician and divine. MD (Oxon Jan. 1745–6), between 1743 and 1763 practised in Northampton. In May 1764 he moved to the rectory of Little Cheverell, near Devizes, Wiltshire.

[4] Possibly, Johann Friedrich Meckel (1724–1774), *Tractatus anatomico physiologicus de quinto pare nervorum cerebri*, Göttingen, A. Vandenhoeck, 1748.

[5] William Hewson (1739–1774), *Experimental inquiries: Part the first. Containing an inquiry into the properties of the blood. With remarks on some of its morbid appearances: and an appendix relating to the discovery of the lymphatic system in birds, fish and animals called amphibious. Part the second. Containing a description of the lymphatic system in the human subject and in other animals. . . . Together with observations*

on the lymph, and the changes which it undergoes in some diseases. Part the third. Containing a description of the red particles of the blood in the human subject and in other animals; with an account of the structure and offices of the lymphatic glands, of the thymus gland, and of the spleen: being the remaining part of the observations and experiments of the late Mr. William Hewson. . . . [Edited] by Magnus Falconar, London, T. Longman, 1772–77.

[6] William Cumberland Cruikshank (1745–1800), *The anatomy of the absorbing vessels of the human body*, London, G. Nicol, 1786.

[7] John Sheldon (1752–1808), *The history of the absorbent system. Part the first. Containing the chylography. . . .* London, printed for the author, 1784.

[8] Benjamin Bell (1749–1806), *A system of surgery*, 6 vols., Edinburgh, C. Elliot, 1783–88.

[9] Albrecht von Haller, *A dissertation on the sensible and irritable parts of animals*, London, J. Nourse, 1755.

[10] Fothergill is demonstrating his allegiance to William Cullen's teaching here as he does in many other places. Cullen (along with other Edinburgh teachers) contested Haller's view that irritability was an autonomous property of muscle, teaching that it was dependent on nervous energy, which in turn, he speculated, was produced by an aerial fluid. See Christopher Lawrence, 'The nervous system and society in the Scottish Enlightenment', in Barry Barnes and Steven Shapin (eds.), *Natural order: historical studies of scientific culture*, Beverly Hills, Sage Publications, 1979, pp. 19–40; J. R. R. Christie, 'Ether and the science of chemistry', in G. N. Cantor and M. J. S. Hodge (eds.), *Conceptions of ether: studies in the history of ether theories 1740–1900*, Cambridge University Press, 1981, pp. 85–110.

[11] Bernhard Siegfried Albinus, *Tables of the skeleton and muscles of the human body . . . Translated from the Latin*, Edinburgh, printed by Balfour and Smellie, for Andrew Bell, engraver, 1777. The subtitle for the second part is dated 1778. Andrew Bell (1726–1809) was an Edinburgh engraver. This edition was reissued as part of Andrew Bell, *Anatomia Britannica: a system of anatomy. Comprising the whole of Albinus's Tables, with selections from Cowper, and other eminent anatomists; illustrated by 109 copper plates. . . . In three parts*, 2 vols. in 1, Edinburgh, A. Bell, 1798.

[12] Alexander Monro, *secundus* (1733–1817), *Observations on the structure and functions of the nervous system*, Edinburgh, William Creech and T. Cadell, 1783; idem, *The structure and physiology of fishes explained and compared with those of man and other animals*, Edinburgh, C. Elliot, 1785.

[13] John Moore (1729–1802), physician and author, MD (Glasgow 1770), *Medical sketches*, London, A. Strahan & T. Cadell, 1786. See next letter.

N° 9 **9**

Bath Octr 13th 1790

Many thanks, kind sir, for your very polite and obliging letter, replete with shrewd observ^s on a variety of subjects, w^h at present I can only acknowledge, not answer by entering into particulars, as I cou'd wish. Your progress in y^r studies affords me the highest satisfaction, but let not your ardour exceed the rules of discretion or interfere with the necess^y hours of sleep and bodily exercise. The mental complacency and even delight which you experience in the prosecution of your studies augurs well and doubtless renders you more able to pursue your inquiries with perseverance and alacrity, but yet still the human machine demands due intervals of rest and relaxation without which all ye mental and corporeal functions languish and disease follows. "Neque semper arcum tendit Apollo."[1] Please to give Moore's Sketches another perusal before you return the book, and as you have read ye 2nd vol. Mem^s of London Medical Soc^y[2] you shou'd, methinks, tho' somewhat prematurely, read ye first now sent with this and a huge catalogue of Lackington's,[3] w^h I have borrowed at Ball's Lib^y[4] till next week, that you may run over and mark out such books as you may soon want, but without ordering them till I see whether they are not some of them in my collections. The books in general are cheaper than in any wholesale catalogue I know, but whether he is the cheapest bookseller in Europe I must leave the literati to judge.

I have only the first edit^{n} of Cullen's Physiol^{ogy}[5] or would send it with this, as you are now well prepared for it. Books in many vols. are perhaps best bo^{t} in sheets or boards, as 2 vol^{s} may often be thrown into one. When you have finished y^{r} pres^{t} reading you may have Hewson. Your letter tho' very long contains no mater^{l} slips worth noticing, except the want of note of interrogation (?) when you ask the question, and the omission of a letter now and then—thro' hurry. Nauseating med^{s} as ipecacuanha, in small doses excite absorption, the digitalis possesses this power in common with the rest, but has also a deleterious quality w^{h} affects the whole genus nervosum in a superior degree, and therefore requires no small caution. Dr Withering[6] asserts that it answers best when given so as to occasion sickness, if so, the above idea is erroneous what you say of its modus operandi. But this requires further observ^{n} and inquiry. Many things he seems to have advanced too hastily and too peremptorily. I am sorry I have got but one of your books looked over, but will glance over the rest as opport^{s} offer. I wish this may be in time for carrier, Dear Sir, y^{rs} assuredly

A. Fothergill

1 "Nor does Apollo always bend his bow". Horace, *Odes*, 2.10.19–20.

2 *Memoirs of the Medical Society of London instituted in the year 1773*, vols. 1–6, London, 1787–1805.

3 Lackington, Allen & Company of London, purported to be the largest and most inexpensive second-hand booksellers in the country. Founded by James Lackington (1746–1815).

4 Ball or Bull equally likely.

5 William Cullen, *Institutions of medicine. Part 1. Physiology*, Edinburgh, 1772. Fourth edition, 1788.

6 William Withering (1741–1799), MD (Edinburgh 1766), practised in Birmingham, member of the Lunar Society, and author of *Account of the Fox-glove, and some of its medical uses: with practical remarks on dropsy and other diseases*, Birmingham, G. G. J. and J. Robinson, 1785.

N° 10 **10**

Bath Novr 24th 1790

Dear Sir,

Various engagements obliged me to postpone answering your last very obliging letter till now, and even now I am pressed for time too much to notice all ye particulars in it, and also in your former letter. Suffice it to say that some extracts from your letters were conveyed to my friend Dr Hawes in London who approved of them so much as to read them to the Med^{l} Soc^{y},[1] consisting of many able judges and that they were very graciously received and met with merited approbation. The gum kino[2] is a powerful antiseptic, at least out of the body, but I have no experience of it in putrid fevers or sore throats. The digitalis I conceive does not act first on the sensorium, but on the nerves of the stomach from whence its action is propag^{d} to the sensorium and from thence to ye rest of the nervous system. In ecchymoses from violent contusions, red blood is undoubtedly extravasated but by suitable discutient applications may be reabsorbed by the adjacent lymphatics. Preparations of lead are powerful remedies to alloy inflammation and pain in recent injuries, but beware of their use where the skin is stripped off; see my Cautions on Lead.[3] Perfectly just is y^{r} observ^{n}—"that an early and guarded education is the bes^{t} security of virtue" etc., and I trust you will experience this in every future stage of your life in the amplest manner. Dr Stonhouse, I have the pleasure to assure you is so much recovered as to be able to preach. He was formerly as eminent in physic as latterly in pulpit eloquence.

No med^l^ books of Dr Moore have come to my knowledge but the Sketches. His tours in France, Italy and Switzerland are well written and his Obser^s^ on men and manners, in general very just, as well as entertaining.[4] I have seen none of the authors on the lymph^s^ you mention. Cruikshank's new edit^n^ is the latest and I imagine the best in the English language, as he had before him my friend Hewson's excellent work in 3 Vol^s^ containing many discoveries w^h^ you are now able to enter upon, and which I send for your perusal and am sorry I have not Cruikshank's to accompany or follow it, nor the new edit^n^ of Cullen's Physiology which will next come in play. But meddle not yet with the materia medica. Remember too many irons in the fire etc. You know the rest. Revise and digest what you have already read, and then I can furnish you in due time with almost the whole of the books you have remarked in Lackington's catalogue, except Hunter[5] and Ferguson[6] neither of which are wanted at present. Gregory[7] and van Swieten[8] tho excellent are premature. Begin not the column of science at the apex, but at the base. Slight serous discharges from the ears are only increased secretion and want of absorption—but real abscesses occur and where the member tympanic is ulcerated then an incurable deafness commonly succeeds. Your mother's I hope is not of this kind but more of this when I next see you. Meanwhile accept my thanks for ye 6 vol^s^ of books herewith returned and w^h^ I have dipped into in various places with satisfaction. Knox[9] seems to merit a place on the same shelf with ye World, the Adventurer and ye Observer, tho' inferior to ye Spectator, Tatler and Guardian. Martin is clear plain and perspicuous. Nicholson is deep in the latest discoveries, a masterly compendium but too abstruse for a beginner, and too superficial for an adept. Simmons[10] seems tolerably accurate, but little more than a large syllabus for lectures, too short as a compendium. Sea bathing by no means to be depended on against canine madness.[11] Aitkin's book[12] will not be necessary. Having thus noticed the principal parts of your last letters, I have but just room to add a nod of hearty approbation on y^r^ rapid progress and to wish you health to proceed. Vale!
A. Fothergill

[1] The Medical Society of London, founded by John Coakley Lettsom (1744–1815) in 1773.

[2] A resin from the Gambia, gum kino, gumm Gambiense, see Royal College of Physicians of London, *The new pharmacopoeia . . . translated . . . by Thomas Healde*, 2nd ed., London, J. W. Galabin, 1788, p. 21.

[3] Fothergill, letter **6**, note 6.

[4] John Moore, *A view of society and manners in France, Switzerland, and Germany . . . By a gentleman who resided several years in those countries,* London, 1779, seventh edition, 1789; and, idem, *A view of society and manners in Italy: with anecdotes relating to some eminent characters*, 2 vols., London, W. Strahan & T. Cadell, 1781. Both books went through numerous editions. Moore graduated MD at Glasgow in 1770.

[5] Presumably a work by either William Hunter (1718–1783) or John Hunter (1728–1793). Probably John. See letter **15**.

[6] Presumably one of the works of James Ferguson, see letter **5**, note 5.

[7] Presumably one of the many editions of James Gregory (1753–1821), *Conspectus medicinae theoreticae*, Edinburgh, Balfour & Smellie, 1780.

[8] Possibly, Gerhard van Swieten (1700–1772), *Commentaria in Hermanni Boerhaave aphorismos de cognoscendis et curandis morbis*, 10 vols., Naples, J. Ponzellius & Manfredi, 1745–1772. Many subsequent editions and English translations.

[9] Unclear reference. Possibly, William Knox (1732–1810), pamphleteer and loyalist during the American Revolution. Under-secretary of state for America 1770–1782.

[10] Samuel Foart Simmons (1750–1813), physician (doctor of physic, Leyden 1776), FRS, author of *Anatomy of the human body*, vol. 1, London, printed for J. Murray, 1780. Simmons translated and edited Claude Person (d. 1758), *Elements of anatomy*, London, 1775; second edition, London, printed for J. Wilkie, 1781.

[11] For an example of the use of sea bathing for rabies see R. James, *A treatise on canine madness*, London, printed for J. Newbery, 1760.

[12] Probably, John Aitkin (d. 1790), *Principles of anatomy and physiology*, 2 vols., London, J. Murray, 1786. Also the author of *Systematic elements of the theory and practice of surgery*, Edinburgh, W. Gordon & W. Creech, 1779. It was no doubt the former work to which Fothergill referred.

N° 12 **11**

Bath Decr 20th 1790

Yesterday, Kind Sir, I was favoured with your good mother's very obliging present of a fine turkey accompanied by your polite letter, for both of which I take the earliest opportunity of returning my sincere thanks. But with all I must request you to convince your dear mother that this kind work is to me a work of supererogation and that this tribute of gratitude was not meant to be exacted at her hands. All your letters breathe the language of a heart overflowing with grateful sensibility, therefore no other visible pledge of your gratitude was necessary. For this with me surpasses every other. But this it seems does not come up to your kind mother's ideas, therefore she must be allowed to go on in her own way as I find nothing short of that will satisfy her. The passages selected from your letter are marked out by Dr Hawes which on looking them over again I find needed no correction, and were such as cou'd only confer credit on the writer. My time at present will but just allow me to notice a few of the principal parts of your present letter now before me. Respiration, tho' of late explained with much ingenuity, does not yet seem to be completely understood. Tho' nitre itself is not present in the atmosphere, yet dephlog^d air, one at least of the constituent principles of the nitrous acid, is always present, and this I take to be quite sufficient to give a florid redness to the blood. As to the phlogis^n so much spoken of, its very existence is called into question by some of the most expert chemists abroad, and all the phenomena are well explained without it. Therefore till its identity is better established Dr Priestley's conclusions concerning respiration etc. must remain sub judice. Nor can animal heat be truly explained on attrition of the principles of the blood or between the blood and the sides of ye arteries. No attrition of fluid parts or of fluids against solids is capable of generating a heat of 96° or 97°, the animal heat. Nor can I allow that the heat of the body always keeps pace with the velocity of the circulation or the vicinity of the heart. Examine by the thermometer the heat of a child whose pulse beats 120 in a minute, and that of an elderly person whose pulse does not exceed 60 or half the above, and I fancy you'll find the temperature in both pretty nearly alike. The same I apprehend wou'd be observed were the instrument placed in the cavity of the heart of an animal and afterwards in the trunk of any large vessel remote from the heart, as the vena porta or iliac vessels, tho' I cannot say I have actually tried the experiment. No sensible or absolute heat or flame can exist, I believe, in nature without dephlogisticated air. By the attraction of this to latent heat a chemical union takes place, and the result is sensible heat, and this I conceive to be the true cause of the heat of animal bodies. But this is connected with some of the most difficult problems in philosophy, and the deepest researches in chemistry, therefore to enter any further into it at present wou'd be premature. Be content at present to investigate the more obvious parts of the animal oeconomy, and leave these subtleties to adepts who, I can assure you, are by no means yet agreed as to the cause of animal heat or of respiration, or even the figure of the red portion of the blood. The tabes mesenterica.[1] when you come to practical authors, you'll find described by Boerhaave,[2] Hoffmann[3] and others; a complaint I believe often fatal to children, and not to be cured unless in the early stage of the disease and before schirrosity or suppuration of the glands takes place. Dr Moore[4] (like many eminent practitioners) who in compliance with popular prejudice, prescribes James's powder, prefers it to emetic tartar as being less emetic, and as more satisfactory to the family, without considering that this is (as you well observe) giving a sanction to empiricism.

Tho' some men of extensive knowledge have become deists, yet none but shallow minute philosophers have ever become atheists, and these I believe very rare, and only so by fits and starts. The most profound philosophers of this or any other country have been Christians by conviction, such as Bacon, Boyle, Locke, Clarke, Newton, Addison, characters not to be equaled among all the host of modern infidels.

Your retrospective view of books already read will be not only useful but pleasing. It is thus after traveling over variegated landscape, that you place yourself on an eminence and retrace all the principal objects, distinguish the several parts with more accuracy and more fully comprehend the beauties of the whole. Instead of saying I am engaged "with going", it would be more correct to say in going through etc., and instead of "imbues the mind with the noblest conceptions" read impresses—and ideas. My tract on lead and copper is not yet published separately and I am sorry.[5] I have not another copy to send you, however I hope Mr Batchelor will recover the one in question for your use. But don't think of buying one. My own copy I expect from Frome in a day or two. You may detain Moore till you have got thro' Hewson, Cruikshank and Cullen. The two former I know are standing pieces. The two latter I expect you'll find so, but can form no judgment till I see them. Wishing you success in all your literary pursuits, I remain,

Dear Sir, with true
regard, sincerely yours
A. Fothergill

[1] Characterised by fever, emaciation and, at post-mortem, enlarged mesenteric lymph glands. Today most cases would be diagnosed as intestinal tuberculosis.

[2] Hermann Boerhaave (1668–1738), chemist and medical teacher at Leyden. Possibly, one of the many editions of Boerhaave, *Aphorismi de cognoscendis et curandis morbis*, Leyden, J. vander Linden, 1709. Later editions contained extensive commentaries by Gerhard van Swieten See letter **10**, note 8. There were many English editions.

[3] Friedrich Hoffmann (1660–1742), *Medicinae rationalis systematicae*, Halle, 1718–40. An English edition appeared in 1783.

[4] Presumably John Moore. See letter **10**, note 4.

[5] Fothergill, letter **6**, note 6.

N° 13 **12**

[Jan. 1791?][1]

Dear Sir,

On my return just now I have met with 2 discourses written for the Humane Society[2] which perhaps you may want to see and if you have not already read my Hints on Animation, the present copy bound with Dr Hawes's address[3] is much at your service. Dr Cullen's[4] being a facsimile of my own is returned with the above wishing you, Dr Sir, a happy new year.

I am much yours A. Fothergill

Walcot Parade, Tuesday Evening

P.S. Wed. noon—The enclosed has waited till now that I forward it by my patient Mr Jenkins of Farleigh Castle, whose wife was no sooner cured of a confirmed dropsy, than the poor man fell into the same deplorable disease accompanied by asthma. This singularly curious explanation of Virgil's Eclogues has just cast up among my books, and as it may be of use to you in your grammatical pursuits it is much at your service. As soon as you can find a leisure day, and can be spared from home come over and breakfast with me at 9 or dine at three. In the interim drop me a line and believe me, Dr Sir, yours assuredly

A. Fothergill

[1] Undated, but the reference to *Hints* (sent June 1790, see letter **6**), the original numbering and "happy new year" suggest early 1791.

[2] Not identified.

[3] See letter **6**, note 7.

[4] The reference is unclear. William Cullen did publish *A letter to Lord Cathcart . . . concerning the recovery of persons drowned and seemingly dead*, London, J. Murray, 1776.

N° 11 **13**

Bath April 9th 1791

My Dear Sir,

Various engag[ts] which would be too tedious to enumerate have obliged me to defer writing, till now that I find myself at length indebted to you for two very kind and very elaborate letters. In both of which I observe with pleasure very evident marks of improvement, and that the outlines of study which at different times I have endeav[d] to sketch out to you have been observed with no small attention. You have already obtained a just idea of the structure and organization of y[r] vernacular language, and have not studied Lowth in vain. The elegancies and final polish will be acquired in due time from Sheridan on Elocution[1] Professor Blair's Lectures on Rhetoric and a perusal of the best English writers, as the Spectator, Tatler, Guardian, Adventurer, Rambler, etc. all which may be considered as classical writers. But these must only be dipped into occasionally as a relief to y[e] mind from severer studies. Please to attend to punctuation, and ye proper use of capitals, circumstances too much neglected by many writers, and yet highly necessary to perspicuity and precision. As to emphasis and pronunciation, I take Sheridan's Dict^{y}[2] to be the best guide. Walker's Dict^{y},[3] price 1 G. just published, is, however, highly extolled in the last Critical Review and may possibly be an improvement on Sheridan. But these in reversion—at present you must complete yourself in the elem^{ts} of medical science. Ornamental accomplishments will afterwards follow in due course. As to anatomy and natural phil^{y} I question whether you can proceed much further till you attend demonstrations and exp^{s}—then Pemberton and M^{ac}laurin on Sir I. Newton's Phil^{y} will come in play. At present you must strive to obtain ye first rudiments of chemistry and ye materia medica. As to ye former there are many elem^{y} books, but I know none more clear and perspicuous for a learner than M^{ac}quer's Elemt^{s} in 2 vol^{s}[4] and also Pemberton's Chemistry[5] both which I can lend you, together with Professor Bergman's Chemical Essays,[6] tho' I have not his work on elective attractions. In the materia medica Dr Cullen's is the best English system but the new edit^{n} is augmented to 2 vol^{s} 4to.[7] Cartheuser,[8] Bergius[9] and Murray[10] on materia medica being in Latin you cannot meddle with these, nor sundry other late valuable authors in different branches without further progress in that language. Therefore if you spare only a single hour a day in the Latin grammar and translating etc. ye time wou'd be well employed.

But I fear too much work is cut out for you already, considering that your master's business must be first attended to. However by oeconomy of time and method in study you'll be advancing by degrees, and when you have once got over the thorny brakes and rugged cliffs w^{h} lead to the hill of licence you'll find the path more smooth and easy, and new, and delightful prospects will begin to open on all hands. Meanwhile you'll keep a steady eye on the motto, "Nil tam difficile est quod non solertia vincat."[11] I shall exercise you a little in Latin by adding a scrap from Dr Hewson's late letter[12] concerning a certain medical élève, whose name I leave you to guess. "Legi maxima voluptate observationes optimi juvenis (de quo omnia sperare licet) acumine et notitia insignitas."[13]

I have glanced over Simmons's and Cruikshank's publications and think both may be useful in your anatomical inquiries, particularly the latter which contains some beautiful (and I believe accurate delineations) of the absorbent vessels, a very important part of anatomy. These with the books above mentioned shall be delivered to your order. Monro's Works, I have not yet got looked over; but hope to do so soon. My respects to your kind mother and acquaint her, and Mr Batchelor, that I hope nothing will prevent the pleasure w^{h} I promise myself from your proposed visit on Thursday next at 3 o'clock over a joint of meat and pudding. As I have not time or room to advert to all particulars in your two long letters, please to note down any inquiries you wish me to reply to against that day and remind me also of the books above mentioned. In the interim I remain, Dr Sir, much y^{rs}

A. Fothergill

P.S. My respects to Mr Palmer am glad to hear he is better, but he must pursue the antiseptic plan longer and be circumspect in his regimen. If he can make it convenient to accompany you on Thursday I shall be glad to see him.

[1] Thomas Sheridan (1719–1788), *A course of lectures on elocution: together with two dissertations on language and some other tracts relative to those subjects*, London, 1762.

[2] Idem, *A general dictionary of the English language*, 2 vols., London, 1780; or the revised and enlarged

edition, *A complete dictionary of the English language, both with regard to sound and meaning,* London, 1789.

[3] John Walker (1732–1807), *A critical pronouncing dictionary and expositor of the English language*, London, 1791.

[4] Pierre Joseph Macquer (1718–1784), *Elements of the theory and practice of chymistry. Translated [by Andrew Reid]*, 2 vols., London, A. Millar & J. Nourse, 1758.

[5] Henry Pemberton, *A course of chemistry, divided into twenty-four lectures, formerly given by . . . Doctor Henry Pemberton, . . . now first published from the author's manuscript, by James Wilson,* London, J. Nourse, 1771.

[6] Torbern Olaf Bergman (1735–1784), *Physical and chemical essays: translated from the original Latin . . . by Edmund Cullen. . . . To which are added notes and illustrations, by the translator [and Thomas Beddoes*], 2 vols., London, J. Murray, 1784; or, 3 vols., London, J. Murray, 1788–91. Fothergill was referring to the latter edition, see letter **15**.

[7] William Cullen, *Lectures on the materia medica*, London, T. Lowndes, 1773; and *A Treatise of the materia medica*, 2 vols., Edinburgh, C. Elliot, London, C. Elliot & T. Kay, 1789.

[8] One of the many editions of Johann Friedrich Cartheuser (1704–1777), *Fundamenta materiae medicae, tam generalis quam specialis in usum academicum conscripta*, 2 vols. in 1, Frankfurt-on-Oder, J. C. Kleyb, 1749–50.

[9] One of the many editions of Peter Jonas Bergius (1730–1790), *Materia medica e regno vegetabili, sistens simplicia officinalia, pariter atque culinaria. Secundum systema sexuale, ex autopsia et experientia*, 2 vols., Stockholm, P. Hesselberg, 1778.

[10] Johan Anders Murray (1740–1791), *Apparatus medicaminum tam simplicium quam praeparatorum et compositorum in praxeos adjumentum consideratus*, Göttingen, J. C. Dieterich, 1776–92.

[11] "There is no difficulty so great that ingenuity does not overcome it". Known proverb. See letter **5**.

[12] Unclear reference.

[13] "I have read with the greatest pleasure the observations of the excellent young man (concerning whom we may hope for everything). Observations which are distinguished by their acuity and insight".

[14] Presumably Alexander Monro, *primus*, *The works of Alexander Monro published by his son, Alexander Monro. . . . To which is prefixed, the life of the author [by D. Monro]*, Edinburgh, C. Elliot, 1781.

N° 14 **14**

Bath June 10th 1791

Dear Sir,

Your kind letter together with the books and your mother's obliging present all arrived safe, for which please to accept my best thanks. But why continue to put yourselves to this unnecessary expense and trouble in accomplishing works of supererogation? Your former excellent letter ought not to have remained so long unanswered, for notwithstanding the manifold interruptions I meet with, yet I cannot wholly absolve myself of remissness when I look back to the date, and reflect on the pains such an elaborate letter must have cost you! However tho' time, I am sensible, can be but ill-spared from your other unavoidable occupations, and the more profitable pursuit of your studies, yet the labour I see with pleasure is far from being lost. On the contrary it affords a most useful exercise in improving your style, and enabling you to write with elegance and facility, an accomplishment aimed at by many but attained by few. In short I find much to commend and but little to blame. Sometimes thro' haste a note of interrogation or a note of admiration is omitted. Sometimes the style rather too diffuse, but little more practice will lead to conciseness and precision. In medical correspondence it is often desirable to say a great deal in a small compass, but while we attempt to condense our ideas we must beware of obscurity. For perspicuity must never be sacrificed to a mistaken brevity, or like him who attempted to enclose Homer's

Iliad in a nutshell, we shall be obliged to confess "Brevis esse laboro—obscurus fio."[1]

I cannot resist sporting now and then a scrap of Latin by way of exercise—wishing you could spare (tho' I fear you cannot) half an hour in a day for the Latin classics. If the method proposed for your mother on the acoustic instrument enables her to hear better, I shall be much pleased. Her hearing more distinctly in a carriage etc. confirms my idea of the deafness being nearly connected with nervous debility and relaxation of the chorda tympani,[2] and you have explained the reason exactly as I conceive it to be. Has she given electricity a fair trial? The case of catalepsy you mention being very uncommon, were it carefully described at large wou'd merit a place in some periodical work of note. As to luxations,[3] Monro and the last anatomists seem to agree in thinking the ligament is lacerated when the luxation is complete. The treatment as you well observe demands saturnine applications and sometimes venesection and other evacuations. The buffy appearance of the blood too often regulates venesection tho' properly speaking it is by no means a just criterion either as to quantity to be taken, or whether venesection be at all requisite. I cou'd say much on this subject but have not leisure now. Tho' the enamel of teeth seems not to be vascular, yet the bony part is. The portrait of Cullen[4] exhibits something of the contours of the features but wants animation and gives a wrong idea. Have heard nothing of Bell's plates.[5] I have more than once seen milky blood but incline to attribute it to unassimilated chyle, not fat with Hewson. The delicate texture of the lungs and the quantity of blood rapidly conveyed thro' that organ demands uncommon discernment in treating pulmonary diseases. I have wrote for young Whittington and he is somewhat better. Notwithstanding some engagements Tuesday, yet I shall be happy to see you and y[r] brother between 5 and 6 over a cup of tea. Till then I must reserve the sequel of the letters and book affairs etc. I have at length glanced over y[r] volumes and will pack 'em up with some of Bergman's works against you come. Meanwhile, remain

D[r] Sir much y[rs]
A. Fothergill

[1] "I labour to be brief, and make myself obscure". Horace, *Art of poetry*, 25–6.

[2] The chorda tympani which crosses the tympanic cavity was described by eighteenth-century anatomists as a branch of the fifth cranial nerve. See Alexander Monro, 'Remarks on the articulation, muscles, and luxation of the lower jaw', in Monro, letter **13**, note 14, pp. 231–80, especially pp. 244–8. It is currently regarded as a branch of the seventh or facial nerve.

[3] A luxation is a dislocation. The jaw was probably being discussed. See ibid., although there is no mention of a lacerated ligament, only a wounded tendon, p. 243.

[4] Not identified.

[5] Bell, letter **8**, note 11.

N[o] 15 **15**

Bath June 15th 1791

Dear Sir,

Herewith I forward your books viz. Monro's works and portrait with Hunter's Animal Oeconomy[1] with thanks, and with the above Bergman's 3 vols. all which I hope you'll receive safe and may keep mine till you start for Edinburgh and also D[r] Hawes's new reports of the Humane Society,[2] Scheele[3] and the Annals of Chemistry,[4] a new periodical work you'll see at Edinburgh. You need not carry many books with you, the carriage of which is very expensive to and fro, and they are generally injured. When you take notes at lectures write in large open lines to fill up in a legible way when you return. This will spare transcribing which is loss of time. Avoid all public amusements and dissipated company which will rob you of that time which may be better employed and lead you into unnecessary expense. Once or twice to the theatre or a concert will be sufficient to gratify your curiosity. Rise early and take time by the forelock, and be early at lectures to get a good place especially at the anatomical theatre, or operations at the Infirmary, or in chemistry. But I need not enlarge on these topics which your good sense and discretion will, I am persuaded, point out to you. But amidst the allurements that will surround, it will require no small resolution to be sufficiently on your guard, and to withstand temptation.

"Nemo mortalium omnibus horis sapit."[5]

Be firm in resolution but without austerity or incivility. "Suaviter in modo sed fortiter in re."[6]

Cultivate acquaintance with senior students of a sedate cast, and gain if possible the favour of the professors, and perhaps they may at last recommend you by letter to some leading men of the faculty in London which may be of real service to you hereafter. Theses are given away at graduations, collect as many as you can—the author is flattered by a polite card requesting one tho' no acquaintance. Strive to get to be a member of the medical societies as soon as you can, by being first a visitor, and attend closely to their debates and note down every new and valuable observation. Preserve this letter as a memento from, Dear Sir, your sincere well-wisher.

A. Fothergill

[1] Monro, letter **13**, note 14, did include a portrait. John Hunter, *Observations on certain parts of the animal oeconomy*, London, [The author], 1786.

[2] William Hawes, *Reports of the [Royal Humane] Society for the recovery of persons apparently drowned*, London, 1779–1789.

[3] Carl Wilhelm Scheele (1742–1786), *The chemical essays of C. W. Scheele, translated from the Transactions of the Academy of Sciences at Stockholm, with additions. [By Thomas Beddoes]*, London, 1786.

[4] Possibly, *Annales de chimie*, 36 vols. in 18, Paris, 1789–1800.

[5] "No mortal shows good sense on all occasions". Known saying.

[6] "Gentle in manner, but resolute in deed". Not attributable.

N° 16 **16**

Bath July 7th 1791

Dear Sir,

At length having obtained a little respite, I hasten to answer the most important parts of your last obliging letter fraught with various observations, and queries on various subjects. Having lately heard that Mr Seagram[1] of Warminster wants an assistant, I have written to the friend of the young man in Northhamptonshire to treat on that subject, but have not heard the result. Shou'd they not agree, I shall advise them to apply (as you properly observe) to some of the capital druggists in London, ye centre of intelligence. Your own destination more immediately demands our consideration at present. If your mind is made up on the subject, and views limited to chirurgery, pharmacy, and midwifery, it will reduce your plan of study very considerably, tho' I still think it was right to lay the foundation on an enlarged comprehensive basis. You may now construct it suitably to your intended superstructure, and accommodate it to your finances. I have duly weighed your open candid acc^{t} of your domestic affairs, the difficulties you have had to struggle with, the circumscribed state of your fortune, your future expectancies, and above all your delicate sense of filial duty so properly discharged and so justly due to a tender and affectionate mother. All these considerations unite in convincing me that you have displayed no small share of prudence, good sense, and moderation in your choice, and that by uniting these 3 branches (as you must do if you fix in the country) you will more speedily and more certainly succeed than if you aspired to a doctor's degree. The success of a physic^{n}, as physic is now conducted, is like a lottery where there are almost innumerable blanks to a prize. Medical merit has but small share in securing success and the disappointment falls much heavier than where the candidate sets out in a humbler station. The trappings and accoutrements of the physician at his first setting out are expensive and yet must be supported at all events, because both the great and small vulgar are dazzled with these far more than by his professional abilities, and if the former are wanting or any wanting or any defect in either dress or address visible, they are sure to draw very unfavorable inferences as to all the rest. Men of discernment see the matter in a different light, but these are few, alas too few in number!

"Rari nantes in gurgite vasto." Virgil[2]

With the foundation you have already laid, and with your diligence and application, as the matter now stands, I persuade myself that a single year at Edinburgh will be sufficient to equip you for surgery, pharmacy, and midwifery. The principal objects of your studies will be anatomy and if you can at easy expense get to be a dissecting pupil so much the better, but subjects are scarce, and dear at Edinburgh, much easier had in London. You should attend the Infirmary closely, much cheaper than a London hospital, as 3 G to 20 G![3] You must attend a course of chemistry and materia medica and the clinical lectures. These will I think be sufficient. For if you attempt to add the theory and practice of physic you will have too many irons in the fire, and they will clash with one another, and the former you'll find enough to occupy your whole time. Should you protract your stay part of the summer you may attend midwifery and perhaps botany at leisure. Obtain a list of the Medical Society and get acquainted with the leading members who will introduce you as a visitor, and perhaps put you in the way of being elected. Strive to conciliate their favour over a dish of tea now and then. To be elected wou'd be a great acquisition, and you wou'd profit by their debates, and acquire a facility of speaking in public. A few words more in answer to some of your queries and then I must hasten to conclusion being now past midnight and the eyelids drowsy. 1 Sweat, I consider as an increased perspiration discharged by the same vessels, but more impregnated with saline acrimony as happens when any discharge is considerably increased. 2nd Lentor and viscidity as a cause of disease is an hypothesis nearly out of date.[4] The state of fluids keep pace with the tone of the solids and their deviations are rather consequences than causes of disease. 3rd The brain is the seat of sense, and intellect, but sensibility or sensation is diffused thro' every ramification of the nervous system. 4th Mineral acids in a dilute state, there is reason to believe, enter the blood as well as vegetables. Alkalis enter beyond a doubt. 5th Epilepsy—your remarks correspond with my own observations in general both as to diet and medicine, on the whole mineral tonics seem preferable, the cortex[5] rarely succeeds. Nor can anything else in certain cases—such as that of poor Miss Edwards. Milk is good but sometimes disposes too much to plethora unless diluted. B. Robinson is an ingenious writer,[6] but fanciful, and too fond of theory, bold in hazarding doubtful remedies, as emetics in hæmoptoe etc. I am glad the books reached you safe. I ordered my servant to pay ye carrier, but not finding him, the shopman also not seeing him, sent the parcel by chaiseman who erased (for prudential reasons) "carriage paid" which ought not to have been done. I am glad cousin B[ainbridge] is better—my respects when you see him, and in the interim forward the enclosed. Take your own time with Bergman, and I can supply you with Lavoisier's Chemistry by Henry[7] and Dr Percival's[8] works etc. Dear Sir,

much yours,
A. Fothergill

[1] Possibly one of two surgeons practising in Warminster, Wiltshire, John Seagram (*fl.* 1760–1800) or Thomas Seagram (1720–1805?). See Wallis and Wallis, letter **1**, note 2, p. 531.

[2] "A few swimmers here and there in the vast sea". Virgil, *Aeneid*, 1.118.

[3] Fothergill was correct. On Edinburgh Infirmary "tickets" see A. Logan Turner, *Story of a great hospital: the Royal Infirmary of Edinburgh*, Edinburgh, Oliver and Boyd, 1937, ch. 9. On London prices see Susan C. Lawrence, *Charitable knowledge: hospital pupils and practitioners in eighteenth-century London*, Cambridge University Press, 1996, p. 108.

[4] Fothergill was again being faithful to Cullen, who had rejected Boerhaave's theory of "lentor". See William Cullen, *The works of William Cullen, M.D.*, 2 vols., Edinburgh, William Blackwood, 1827, vol. 2, p. 491.

[5] Cortex Peruvianus, cinchona or Peruvian bark.

[6] Bryan Robinson (1680–1754), physician and mathematical writer, MD (Trinity College, Dublin), after 1745 professor of physic, member of the Irish Royal College of Surgeons, and three times president of the King and Queen's College of Physicians in Ireland.

[7] Antoine Laurent Lavoisier (1743–1794), *Essays on the effects produced by various processes on atmospheric air; with a particular view to an investigation of the constitution of the acids, . . . translated from the French by Thomas Henry*, Warrington, 1783.

[8] Thomas Percival (1740–1804), *Essays, medical, philosophical, and experimental*, London, 1767. Fourth edition, 1788–89.

No 17 **17**

Bath August 6th 1791

Accept, my dear sir, in answer to your long and very obliging letter a short hasty reply which is all that time will allow at present. My design was to have called on you and also my cousin Bainbridge in the course of this week, but some new arrivals, and other indispensable engagements have defeated my purpose. However as you promise me a visit on Monday he will probably accompany you if you let him know tomorrow (Sunday).[1] If the day is favourable I shall hope to see you here by two o'clock to partake of a joint of mutton. If you ride, order my servant to put your horses in my stable and enter no inn but mine at the sign of 107 miles from London wh you'll find engraven on stone near my lower door.

Dr Gregory's Duties of a Physician merits your reperusal again and again whether you put on the Togam medicam or not.

"Nocturna versate manu, versate diurna" Hor[2]

After a regular course you'll comprehend Bergman tho' the new nomenclature renders it a puzzle till the terms become familiar.[3] Angiology and neurology can only be acquired by demonstration on the recent subject, and by proper preparations, all w^{h} you'll see in abundance at Profess^{r} Monro's theatre, and afterwards at Dr Hunter's excellent Museum in Windmill Street, w^{h} is perhaps the first collection of anatomical preparations in Europe.[4] That of ye present John Hunter is, I am informed, the next.[5] Now a word or 2 in ans^{r} to y^{r} queries and then conclude. 1 Notwithstanding the vain boasting of quacks concerning their infallible solvents, I believe no such thing as a safe and certain solvent of ye stone in ye bladder is yet known. The mephitic water is perfectly safe, affords relief and prevents accretion and perhaps approaches nearer to the grand desideratum than anything yet discovered. But I cannot presume to call it a certain solvent. Those who pretend it does not act as a diuretic, are deceived, and their writings mislead the public as I can prove from long and attentive observation. 2^{d} Emetics in the phthysis pulmonalis are strongly insisted on by my friend Dr Reid whose book[6] I will lend you on y^{r} return, but tho' the practice in certain cases is doubtless beneficial yet in others it is doubtful, if not injurious, especially where there is hæmoptysis. 3rd Some attribute the vermifuge power of [?] Stan[. . .] to an arsen[ical][7] principle, but so volatile a substance as arsenic if present must be dissipated by the melting [of] the tin. I conclude its action is mechanical, and that the filings are the best pp^{n}. 4 If the headache proceeds from sympathy with the stomach in consequence of vit^{d} bile or indigestion, the speediest remedy is an emetic followed by repeated doses of calcined magnesia and copious dilution. To prevent a return, tonics, bitters and aromatics will succeed, if temperance be observed, otherwise not. Coffee affords temp^{y} relief.

5 The modus operandi of medicine is still imperfectly understood. Their act^{n} on ye blood is I think evidently in a secondary way.

The chief action is on the nerves of the stomach and intestines. No direct proof that bark or steel enter proprio marte[8] the lacteals, yet the chyle imbued with virtues probably finds entrance in a superior degree to what modern physiologists are disposed to allow. Besides the ærial fluids evolved may produce new combinations at present little dreamt of even by our most enlightened pneumatic philosophers. More when we meet. Thanks for Cullen's M.S.[?] which shall be taken care of till your return. I hope you'll receive this today, and am, Dear Sir, yours assuredly

A. Fothergill

[1] The date of the letter is probably correct. Sunday was the 7th in 1791.

[2] "Thumb their pages by night, thumb them by day". Horace, *Art of poetry*, 269.

[3] I.e. Lavoisier's new chemical nomenclature.

[4] William Hunter's museum was in Great Windmill Street, London.

[5] John Hunter's museum was in Castle Street, London.

[6] Thomas Reid (1739–1802), *An essay on the nature and cure of phthisis pulmonalis*, London, 1782; idem, *The second edition enlarged. To which is added an appendix on the use and effects of frequent vomits*, London, T. Cadel [*sic*], 1785.

[7] Not all decipherable but the context indicates powdered tin—Stanni pulvis—which was used as a vermifuge.

[8] "By his own courage," or, as here, "by its own powers". Ovid, *Letters from Pontus*, 4.7.14.

N° 18 **18**

Bath August 10th/91

My Dear Sir,

On reconsideration, Blanchard's Lexicon Technicum[1] being in Latin and that not very perspicuous, I fear it wou'd not answer so well as Motherby's Dictionary[2] therefore have not sent it but you shall have it if you choose. If you cannot get books regul[y] f[m] the College Lib[y], by subscribing to some medical circulating Lib[y] you'll get supplied so as to avoid the carriage of many books backwards and forwards w[h] is very expensive. The enclosed introductory letters require only a wafer[3] before you deliver them. I hope they may in some measure answer the intentions for which they are intended, tho' you'll find the professors at first a little reserved, as it becomes them to avoid showing open partiality to any one, however warmly recommended. Old Monro[4] and Cullen alas are gone, with them I had interest, tho' little with the present set. They were the open patrons of rising merit. I know Duncan[5] but little, Hamilton[6] still less. Shou'd they prove very civil and attentive to my request drop them a short polite note of acknowledgement. This will conciliate favour and enable you to ask a question when at a loss and they will like you the better for it. As to dress—let it be plain neat and becoming a student—black used to be a favourite and fashionable dress and at the same time frugal. Any thing tawdry or coxcombical disgusts the professors. Snuff taking is but too fashionable. I found it contagious and contracted a bad habit which I have never been able to leave off—you may take a pinch if asked but never carry a box—if you do, you deserve to be boxed. Choose an airy light room with few students in the house. If good Mr Mosman in the Lawn Market be living, call on him with my best respects and grateful remembrance, a worthy obliging man free from pride or ceremony. He may assist you in recommending proper lodgings and prevent imposition. Also M[r] and M[rs] Hart, High Street, my other acquaintance. Except the Miss Crows (Cowgate), to whom my respects, are dead or removed. Be home at your lodgings before 10 at night or you may receive unsavoury offerings from Cloacina f[m] every lofty building.[7] The caddies or ticketed porters[8] are faithful creatures bound to good behaviour and you may send my book or parcel or trunk very safely by them if they wear the ticket. Carry only 30[s] or 40[s] in your pocket, conceal the rest, if in notes, under your garter. Deposit spare cash at some bank where perhaps you may have small interest as 2 or 3 percent as at Bath, rather than keep it in their bureaus[9] to w[h] they may have more than one key. Let not the smiling Scotch lassies inveigle you into intrigue much less matrimony which they are ever on the watch to do and may easily bring about as in joke with unwary youths—but sometimes. "Hæ nugæ seria ducent in mala."[10] I remember 2 or 3 such matches. Keep a little journal of occurrences, and a regular account of disbursements, and if you should fall short of a little cash now, or hereafter, and your poor mother be straitened as to a remittance, let me know. The above hints tho' seemingly trivial may prove of material use to you, and had I been thus admonished beforehand some money and much time would have been saved. Before you return, and after the lectures are over, it may not be amiss to make a short excursion of 2 days to see Stirling, Glasgow etc. I cannot recollect anything material further at present, but let me hear from you at least once more before you start for the land of cakes, where as Virgil observes on another occasion!!

"Infelix lolium et steriles dominantur avenae."[11]

But respects to your worthy mother.

Dear Sir, adieu!
A. Fothergill

[1] Probably, Steven Blankaart (Stephanus Blancardus) (1650–1702), *Lexicon medicum renovatum, in quo totius artis medicae termini. . . . exponuntur. . . . Hisce adjungitur Graecarum vocum etymologia; tum earum Belgica, Germanica, Gallica, Anglica &c. interpretatio; cum indicibus. Ed. novissima,* Leyden, S. Luchtmans, 1735.

[2] George Motherby (1732–1793), *A new medical dictionary; or, general repository of physic*, London, J. Johnson, 1775.

[3] A flour and gum mixture used to seal letters.

[4] Alexander Monro, *primus*, professor of anatomy in the university of Edinburgh.

[5] Andrew Duncan, the elder (1744–1828), since 1790 professor of the theory or institutes of medicine in the university of Edinburgh.

[6] Alexander Hamilton (1739–1802), since 1780 professor of midwifery in the university of Edinburgh.

[7] At ten o'clock each evening the day's "domestic abominations" (the "flowers of Edinburgh") were flung into the street. Henry Grey Graham, *The social life of Scotland in the eighteenth century*, 5th ed., London, Adam and Charles Black, 1969, p. 83.

[8] Caddies carried messages and parcels around Edinburgh for a penny. In spite of their poverty they had a reputation for honesty. See Graham, ibid., p. 90.

[9] I.e. at his lodgings.

[10] "These frivolities will lead to serious evils". Horace, *Art of poetry*, 451.

[11] "The unfruitful darnel and barren wild oats prevail". Virgil, *Georgics*, 1.154.

N° 19 **19**

Bath Aug[t] 27th 1791

Accept, D[r] Sir, my best thanks for your kind present of a live turkey which struts about my garden and expands its tail with great majesty, unconscious, poor animal, of its impending fate! Reluctant to destroy these poor innocent unoffending creatures, I forbear to pronounce its doom from day to day and to avoid which shall, at last, probably send it to some friend at a distance. Your obliging letter tho' "too civil by half" in overrating my endeavours to serve your interest, yet as it bespeaks a mind overflowing with gratitude, it does no small honour to the head, and heart of the writer, whose language glows with sensibility and is expressed with energy. What I have said in your favour to the professors was not meant as a flattering eulogy, but my real sentiments of your merit, concerning which I am convinced they will not find me mistaken or guilty of drawing an overstrained panegyric, which, I well know, often defeats the author's intention. If D[r] Duncan is now President of the College,[1] as I have since heard, you will alter the direction of my letter accordingly. Since my good neighbour M[r] Dawson[2] returned from Edin[r] I have made particular enquiry as to some points that concern you, and have requested his sentiments in writing, which he has kindly put down at large and which I here enclose. If the weather proves even tolerable, I think you may save much expense in traveling by observing his directions and see the country to great advantage by sitting with the coachman on the box, but on the roof is much easier taking with you a stout great coat to have in readiness in case no room can be had within, in case of rain. Be sure to travel in boots at all events, and when coaches are changed see your luggage replaced yourself. If you have not a leathern portmanteau with lock and key, I can lend you mine, as I don't want it, or saddle bags, both w^h lie idle. Mr D[awson] cou'd learn nothing of Mr Hart or Mr Mosman at $Edin^r$ so I fear they are no more, but Mrs Morison will I trust supply the defect. If they are dead of w^h she will also inform you, as perhaps they have only removed to another quarter. The books you propose are very proper to be reperused before you start. You may omit going further in nat^l philosophy till some short course occurs hereafter from some of the traveling lecturers, which added to your reading will be quite sufficient. Shou'd you have leisure you may now properly look over my namesake's works, which I can lend you. But never more compare to Anthony F^l who shrinks from every comparison of this nature, and who must be content to contemplate his character in awful silence and admiration, and to follow with humble step!—"non passibus æquis."[3] Shou'd you find a want of Dr Cullen's works or any others in your possession or mine you can have them sent by the wagon, but till you find what books are now used in the preliminary way, it will be best to take a few, especially as you have carefully gone thro' them already. Being called to Mr Halliday at Bradford the morning of the thunder storm, I passed thro' Trowbridge, and calling at Mr P[almer] found you was gone as I expected, so passed on to see Bainbridge and being weatherbound at Freshford and Stoke did not reach home till half past 10 in the evening. The flashes of lightning from various parts of the heavens were uncommonly vivid and awfully sublime particularly as I passed over Claverton Down. My Servant who was much frightened kept close behind me, and we fortunately escaped the danger of that tremendous night, w^h spread horror over the greatest part of this island, and much damage in some places I am sorry to find has accrued. Keep a little journal of remarkables in your journey, and afterwards at $Edin^r$, if your poor mother finds any difficulty in raising the necessary supplies and a small sum will prove agreeable, I hope you will make free in mentioning it. To the instructions already offered I see nothing at present to add but what your own good sense will readily suggest. "Nullum numen abest, si sit Prudentia"[4]

Dear Sir, much yours
A. Fothergill

P.S. But respects to y^r D^r mother with many thanks. At my request Mr Dawson will spare you his $Edin^r$ guide till you set out which will give you much information. No such guide in my time. Tempora mutantur[5] apropos. I have just rec^d 2 copies of a new book on animation[6] from Dr Hawes who requests your acceptance of one of them. If you write to him by private hand or under cover to me, he lives in Spital Square now not Bury St. A spare copy of my thesis[7] is just cast up among my Lawtonian collection, and is at y^r service. When y^r classes are over you may by way of exercise in y^r Latinity translate it into English if you should find leisure.

As soon as you can make acquaintance with any of the members of the Royal Society [of Edinburgh] or Royal Medical Society get introduced as a visitor, and you may then present these copies of my tracts to the secretary, and this may tend to increase your acquaintance and render you more welcome at a future visit. In spring you'll learn who are the intended graduates, and by getting acquainted you'll obtain their theses

Vale!

[1] Andrew Duncan, the elder, became President of the Royal College of Physicians of Edinburgh in 1790.
[2] Probably Benjamin Dawson (1750–?), Bath apothecary. See Wallis and Wallis, letter **1**, note 2, p.158. He seemingly lived, as Fothergill did, in Walcot Parade. See letter **53**.
[3] "Not with equal steps", i.e smaller. Virgil, *Aeneid*, 2.724.
[4] "No deity is absent, if there be prudence". Juvenal, *Satires*, 10.365.
[5] "The times are changing". Attributed to Kaiser Lothar I (795–855).
[6] Not identified.
[7] Anthony Fothergill, *De febre intermittente*, Edinburgh, A. Donaldson & J. Reid, 1763.

N° 20 **20**

Bath Oct. 14th 1791

Dear Sir, Yesterday I was fav^d^ with your obliging letter and am glad you had an agreeable journey, arrived safe and met with so favorable a reception from professors to whom my letters were addressed. My wish was that you should be respectfully received at first setting out and have the satisfaction to find this accomplished beyond my expectation. It now remains with you by assiduity and attention, to confirm the favourable impressions, and secure, if possible, their future friendship. From the circumstances you mention and the defalcation already made in y^r^ present cash (w^h^ I make no doubt your poor mother thought a very considerable sum) I foresee you will find some difficulty in raising the necess^y^ supplies, and that it will therefore be absolutely necess^y^ for you to exercise the most rigid oeconomy. However as your views are limited to surgery, pharm^y^ and midwifery, there can be no occasion for y^r^ branching into any material expense beyond that in w^h^ you have already embarked. Indeed the advanced rate of a student's establishment, even in this circumscribed path, forbids all thoughts of it. Your Infir^y^ Ticket extends instead of next Novem^r^ to Novr 1792, or else there is some mistake. Instead of 1 G the even^g^ anatomical demonstr^n^ used only to be 5^s^.[1] The lectures you mention, with the Infirmary and clinical lectures are abundantly sufficient, and more, I fear, than you can find time to digest. The theory of medicine you'll learn from authors, and will have the indic^ns^ and outlines sufficiently delineated from the practical chair. The anatomical professor will give you the basis and principles of surgery, the rest you'll find in practical writers at the Infirmary. Your notes should be full, but rather a neat abridgement than an attempt to grasp at the whole, you may correct and expand on return home, observing to leave sufficient room for interlineations, a good fountain pen may greatly expedite your labour, and save time in taking notes, espec^y^ as you are unacquainted with shorthand. [?] G on introd^n^ to ye Medical Society![2]—This is a new and heavy import unknown in my time. Your time I fear will not admit of entering, not to mention y^r^ finances. If you can obtain admission about once a month as visitor, as seems probable, it may fully answer your purpose as you stay but one session, you must judge for yourself in this matter. One copy of the tract being intended for the Royal Soc^y^ of Edin^r^ and the other for the Royal Medical Soc^y^ you have by mistake given a duplicate to the latter. The Secretary will be so kind as to allow you to rectify this mistake. I called on your brother lately at Bristol and have seen since at Bath, your and all well. Your letters rec^d^—of which I had an agreeable account so be easy on those heads.

Your boarding with M^r^ M^c^auley,[3] a gent of the faculty, was a happy thought and will, I flatter myself, redound greatly to your improvement, and to your information in a variety of interesting particulars. The situation is central, and desirable, and if you can secure the friendship of M^{r} M[^{c}auley] and y^{r} med^{l} colleague of 2 y^{rs} standing, it will, I think, be a great acquisition. Present my respects to these gent_. and acquaint them (if you see proper) with any sentiments on this head. When you meet at meal times, if you hint y^{r} doubts and difficulties they will kindly clear them up, and by instructive conversation you will thus be enabled to fill the interstices of time with mental improvement. "Vita brevis—ars longa"[4] therefore catch time by the forelock. "Nil actum credens dum quid superesset agendum."[5] If on the contrary you should turn idle and neglect instruction, I hope y^{r} comrades will give me notice that we may get you safely lodged in the Toll Booth. The inclosed bank bill will I hope reach you safe, of w^{h} please to enter a memorandum in y^{r} pocket book, and mind to endorse it when you pay it away. Let not letter writing encroach on y^{r} time except on real business, or when a lucky opportunity offers of conveyance by London or otherwise. I value y^{r} last and indeed most of y^{r} letters very highly but must now consider y^{r} silence as an indication of business, and y^{r} time too precious to be squandered in scribbling to, Dear Sir, y^{rs} very

sincerely and affectionately
N.B. Mr Dawson's A. Fothergill
Compts

[1] In 1755 Alexander Monro, *secundus*, employed John Innes as a dissector who oversaw the students who returned in the evening to examine the bodies dissected in the day. In 1777 Andrew Fyfe joined Innes, who died shortly afterwards. Fyfe was still in this post when Woodforde attended the university. See Rex E. Wright-St. Clair, *Doctors Monro: a medical saga*, London, The Wellcome Historical Medical Library, 1964, p. 79.

[2] The figure at [?] looks like a 5 but it cannot be, or it is a mistranscription. When the Society was founded there seems to have been no introduction fee. Members paid sixpence after each weekly meeting to defray expenses. There were fines for absences without reason. See James Gray, *History of the Royal Medical Society* 1737–1937, Edinburgh University Press, 1952, p. 31. Five guineas seems a huge amount. There was an entrance fee of 2 guineas in 1820 but there are no records of earlier financial matters. In 1969 the fee had gone down to 1 guinea. We are grateful to Pat Strong, Permanent Secretary of the RMS, for this information.

[3] Not identified.

[4] "Life is short, art is long". Hippocrates, *Aphorisms*, 1, i.

[5] "Thinking nothing had been done so long as anything remained to be done". Lucan, *Civil War*, 2.657

N° 21 **21**

Bath Feb: 6th 1792

Dear Sir,

Pursuant to y^{r} request respecting the loan of a small sum to subscribe to some additional lectures, I forwarded without delay the middle of Octr last a Bank of England bill of £10 by the post, w^{h} I make no doubt you received safe. Tho' I did not require an immediate answer, nor press you to write often as heretofore for fear of wasting y^{r} time or encroaching on y^{r} studies, yet after so many thoughts have elapsed I cannot but wish to hear that the bill proved a seasonable supply at that juncture, and that you pursue your studies with alacrity and success. To spare you the postage of this I send [it] by Mr Dawson's parcel to M^{r} M^{c}leary, apoth^{y} in Edin^{r}, with whom it perhaps may be not amiss to be acquainted, as professional men who are residents may now and then befriend a stranger without much trouble in a thousand nameless streets. Your quarters where you entered I hope prove agreeable, and that by this time you find yourself at home among the worthy North Britons who, tho' like the English show a little reserve on first acquaintance, yet afterwards, like them, prove steady and sincere friends where they discover signs of merit to attract their attention. It will, however, behove you to use discretion among the numerous acquaintances with whom you may chance to fall in company, how you form friendships which you will find advisable to confine to a select few, whose character and morals will bear a strict scrutiny. And this maxim you will find important not only now, during y^r residence in a strange place, but also in y^r future transactions thro' life wherever your lot may chance to be. Amidst the various deceptions and deep laid artifices to circumvent[1] which are daily had recourse to, especy in populous cities, by deep designing men hackneyed in ye ways of fraud, a literary man, devoted to his books, has but little chance unless perpetually upon his guard. I shou'd not have dwelt so long on this point had I not thought it a matter of consequence, and tho' your own prudence may in some measure have anticipated me, yet in such a world as this, which may be considered as a grand theatre where every species of legerdemain and deception is daily practised by a set of masked characters, inexperienced youth can hardly be too wary. Sæpe numero decipiuntur specie recti.[2] Cautela ergo non nocet![3]

Before Mr Dawson answers M^r M^cleary's order, he wishes to know from you whether he has a good shop and appears to live in credit and in a good situation etc. Messrs Palmer and Silv^r well, when I was there on Wednesday last. Dr Bar [indecipherable] is dead and 3 Candidates enter ye lists. Was called to Mr Edgell butcher at Trowbridge in extremis. Died next morning—after a full season Bath now grows thin among the French nobles. The celebrated Countess Gurlis and her very accomplished pupil the Princess D'Orleans were lately under my care. I have only room to add—I remain,

Dr Sir much y^rs
A. Fothergill

N.B. Shou'd you at any time change y^r lodgings be sure to notice in writing the alteration, at the Post Office.

[1] The sentence makes more sense with "to circumvent" placed after "fraud". Presumably there has been a transcription error of some sort.
[2] "Often we are deceived by a mirage of right". Horace, *Art of poetry*, 25.
[3] "Caution therefore does no harm". Not attributable.

N° 23 **22**

Bath March 15th 1792

Dear Sir

Your very obliging letter of Feb. ult. brought me the welcome tidings of your health and your happy progress in y^r studies, and the seasonable arrival of the bank note, all w^h afforded me much satisfaction. Your strict attention to oeconomy and abstaining from the allurements of the idle, the vicious and the voluptuous will in time amply reward y^{r} self denial, and the interim cannot but prove highly satisfactory to your affectionate mother, whose maternal care and tender solicitude, no doubt follows you in your absence with anxious eye and looks forward with impatience for your joyful return. By steady perseverance in the good course you have begun according to the plan I endeavoured to sketch out for you, I flatter myself you will preserve your health, insure the esteem of your preceptors and obtain an education perfectly adequate to your station, at a moderate expense. But if you once give ear to that Siren pleasure, your declared foe of study and every laudable pursuit, the fertile source of folly, intemperance and disease, farewell of all hopes of excelling in y^{r} profession, or gaining the confidence and good will of mankind! For who would willingly entrust his health to the care of one, who is daily hastening to destroy his own? It is recorded of the sage Ulysses that on his approach to the dangerous coast where the Siren poured forth her songs and blandishments, if he but listened, he knew he should certainly be undone as had many of his predecessors. He therefore wisely stopped both his ears, and ordered his attendants to bind him to the mast. By listening to the Siren how many students of promising abilities have suffered shipwreck at an early period in their fame, health, and fortune, too many instances of which have happened within my own remembrance! "Sperne voluptates: nocet empta dolore voluptas"![1]

The present year I consider as the most important of your life. Ergo, "carpe diem"[2] and "Ito pede certo et securo."[3]

"Nil tam difficile est quod non solertia vincat."[4]

Rise early—study diligently, live temperately, allow 1 hour for exercise, 6 or 7 for repose.

In protracting your stay till $Sept^{r}$ you judge right. Lectures still going on, libraries open, Infirmary with numerous invalids, notes to be revised, in a word the summer may be well employed, no want of work at $Edin^{r}$ to those that are industrious, not even during recess. At present you have many irons in the fire, too many I s^{hd} think for most artists to engage with at once. But knowing your dexterity, I flatter myself you will manage them all well, and not suffer one to burn or calcine, w^{h} however might probably happen were you permitted to give full scope to your propensity to frequently sitting down to write long letters to A.F. when you should be busy at your anvil. If any preliminary directions of mine in conducting y^{r} studies have contributed to enable you now "to feel y^{r}self not inferior to many of y^{r} colleagues of 2 or 3 years standing" I rejoice at it most sincerely and think the labour well bestowed. But however glad I may be to hear of your progress, I must not retard your literary career so honorable to yourself by tempting you to support a too frequent and laborious correspondence. I gladly engage this opportunity by Mr Dawson's packet to the druggist of answering y^{r} last very acceptable letter, and must not forget to present best respects from Mr Batchelor and Bainbridge and Mr Dawson and Dr Hawes. The terms of the Med^{l} Soc^{y} are strangely advanced since my time, and it is now to be regretted, if thro' some narrow policy the door of science is to be shut against young men of genius, and not to be opened unless they are provided with a Golden Key[5] w^{h} may not always be at hand. In this case they certainly have a right to avail themselves of the key of some good natured colleague as often as they decently can, and at other times learn the result of any interesting debate from the Sec^{y} or other members and this may answer y^{e} purpose tolerably well. But had it been mentioned in time y^{e} $Gent^{n}$ alluded to should not have been kept out for want of a G[olden] Key. To the professors who in consequence of my recommendation have shown you so much attention and kindness, be pleased to present my grateful acknowledgements: and it will be your duty and also y^{r} interest to strive earnestly to merit their esteem, and profit by their instructions, of w^{h} indeed you leave me no room to doubt, but have already given me very ample testimony. Attend closely at the Infirmary to ye phenom^{a} of diseases, ye operations of medicines, the effect of external applications, the diet, regimen, oeconomy and ventilation of ye house: of inattention to the last, I think Mr Howard[6] complains. Indeed there are few hospitals or prisons in w^{h} this important circumstance is not still too much neglected. A neglect w^{h}, I am persuaded, often defeats the best concerted plan of treatment. What is all the pomp and parade of med^{s} when compared to ye animated influence of a current of fresh air? In foul offensive wards, nurses and patients often shut windows or air vents that ought to be kept open. If you mark this, complain boldly to the physicians or clinical professor who may be too much engaged to notice every abuse. A lying-in hosp^{l} and another for maniacs will be great acquisitions to the College and to the pupils.[7] A course of clinical lectures on insane subjects wou'd be very interesting to the cause of science and of humanity. Obliged as I often am to write letters by candlelight and at a late hour as at present (1/2 past 1) I feel the inconvenience very sensibly and must request you in future to use blacker ink and larger type. 'Tis a pity such a well—I mean ill-written—letter but replete with elegant phraseology sh^{d} be scarcely legible. Imitate not my minikin microscopical hand w^{h} I hereby prohibit you, and every person from using except—myself. The moment a man begins to use spectacles he is said to be old, but observe tho' it is the ton to be near-sighted, I am not ambitious to wear spectacles or to be thought old, tho' I confess my garrulity in this long letter may seem a prelude towards it. Take care of y^{r} health and of y^{r} sight. Without these, what is knowledge to you, Dr Sir, y^{rs}

A. Fothergill—Adieu!

[1] "Scorn pleasure: pleasure bought with woe does harm". Horace, *Epistolae*, 1.2.55.

[2] "Seize the day". Horace, *Odes*, 1.11.8.

[3] "Go with steady pace and free from care". Not attributable.

[4] "No difficulty is so great that ingenuity does not overcome it". Known proverb, obviously one of Fothergill's favourites; see letters **5** and **13**.

[5] See letter **20**, note 2.

[6] John Howard (1726–1790), advocate for prison reform in Britain and abroad.

[7] A lying-in hospital was erected in 1793. The foundation stone of the Royal Edinburgh Asylum for the Insane was not laid until 1809, although clearly special provision for lunatics had been discussed much earlier. See John D. Comrie, *History of Scottish medicine*, 2 vols., London, The Wellcome Historical Medical Museum, 1932, vol. 2, pp. 455, 465.

N° 22 **23**

Bath April 18th 1792

My dear Sir

Having in my last enlarged on some of the topics w^{h} appeared to me most intimately connected with your present and even future welfare and having at present nothing either new or important to add, I shall confine myself to a few general remarks in ans^{r} to your last very affectionate letter. For I can not let slip so favorable an opportunity of throwing off a few hasty lines (volante calamo)[1] by the Dawsonian packet laden with a cargo of sweets and bound to the barren regions of the north where, if we may believe the great Johnson—"not a bee will grow"—and to which Virgil's description of another dreary spot may seem applicable, where he says—

"Infelix lolium et steriles dominantur avenæ."[2]

Therefore, chameleon like, you must learn to live upon air, and content yourself with intellectual food. But as fasting wonderfully sharpens the senses, and quickens all the mental faculties, I can easily account for the rapid progress you are making in y^{r} studies. Hence perhaps it is that the Scotch people, by dint of meagre diet become as keen as ye northern blast, and excel all other nations in deep speculation. So you must make a virtue of necessity, and as oats are the chief produce of that sterile country, you must content yourself with oaten cake, oatmeal gruel, and now and then (if you can get it) a little oatmeal crowdy.[3] If you but just kept from starving so much the better. You'll return, we expect, as thin as a rat, and with famine in y^{r} countenance, but then you'll return sharp set and with y^{r} senses as keen as a razor. 'Twas by mere dint of starvation that the learned Ty[?][4] became such an adept in the occult sciences, and to prove an overmatch for all the fat fellows of both our universities. The dancing bear could never be brought to move a minuet with such grace and agility were he not kept on very low diet during his education. The little devil, I am told, was an awkward clumsy fellow, till he was starved down to almost a skeleton, w^{h} brought him to such a surprising degree of activity of body and mind as to perform with ease such feats of agility as none, one wou'd think, but the real devil himself wou'd ever be capable of. In short since low diet, or in other words <u>starving</u>, so wonderfully excites all the active faculties of men, of brutes and of devils, it is hoped you will patiently submit to y^{r} fate, and since all's for the best, consider this meagre regimen as not only salutary, but necess^{y} during y^{r} stay.

But now ad rem,[5] and to be serious, as you continue thro' the summer I think it will be right to attend D^{r} H[ome's][6] clin^{l} lect^{s}. Boerhaave, van Swieten and Morgagni,[7] I can lend you on your return. To go thro' them is a work of time. I observe with satisfaction your attention to hosp^{l} cases and the result of the different methods employed in the treatment. The want of success among such learned and able professors may serve to inspire a becoming diffidence in their pupils who on first entering into practice are generally too sanguine and ready on all occasions to pronounce—"Veni, vidi, vici,"[8] forgetting the power of medicine at best is but a relative term. If such profound chemists as Dr Black adopt the Lavoisierian theory ye phlogistic doctrine must, I think, give way.[9] The former from its simplicity and the ingenuity with w^{h} it is supported is truly fascinating. The latter pleads the sanction of time and maintains its ground as a useful auxiliary at a dead lift. The rabies canina has been frequent and fatal in many parts of England. Do you meet with anything new or important in the prevention or cure? Any clin^{l} lectures thereon? or any good remarks in the Encyclopedia Edinb[10] at the College Lib^{y}? Whether I shall find leisure to give a few remarks on that terrible malady in the Bath Soc^{s} next vol.[11] in compliance with ye wish of some of ye members, I am uncertain. The faculty have long been silent, and art seems exhausted. Sh'd you find my friend Mr J^{hn} Mosman still in the land of the living remember kindly to him and believe me, Dr Sir, y^{rs} assuredly

<u>A. Fothergill</u>

PS: Dr Hawes having seen some of your letters has conceived an esteem for the writer, commends his continuance at Edin^r and says everything kind on that head

With Mr Dawson's best thanks etc.

[1] "With flying pen".

[2] "The unfruitful darnel and barren wild oats prevail". Virgil, *Georgics*, 1.154. See letter **18**.

[3] Crowdy, crowdie: porridge.

[4] This word has defied decipherment, being variously read by numerous people as Ty, Pig, Tig, etc. It was probably a reference unknown to the transcriber, but from what follows it would seem to suggest the figure was Sir Isaac Newton (1642–1727), legendary (quite undeservedly) for his neglect of food. See Rob Iliffe, 'Isaac Newton: Lucatello professor of mathematics', in Christopher Lawrence and Steven Shapin (eds.), *Science incarnate: historical embodiments of natural knowledge*, Chicago University Press, 1998, pp. 156–201.

[5] "To the matter in hand".

[6] Francis Home (1719–1813), MD (Edinburgh 1750), since 1768 professor of materia medica in the university of Edinburgh.

[7] Giovanni Battista Morgagni (1682–1771), *The seats and causes of diseases investigated by anatomy. . . . Translated from the Latin . . . by Benjamin Alexander*, 3 vols., London, A. Millar & T. Cadell, 1769.

[8] "I came, I saw, I conquered". Suetonius, *Caesar*, 37.

[9] Joseph Black had definitively adopted Lavoisier's chemistry by 1790. See R. G. W. Anderson, *The Playfair collection and the teaching of chemistry at the University of Edinburgh*, 1713–1858, Edinburgh, The Royal Scottish Museum, 1978, p. 26.

[10] Possibly, *Encyclopedia Britannica*, Edinburgh, A. Bell and C. Macfarquhar, 1771. Second edition, 1778–83.

[11] Anthony Fothergill, *Essay on the nature of the disease occasioned by the bite of a mad dog. . . . To which is prefixed, a letter to the author from the Count L. de Berchtold, on the efficacy of olive oil.* [Bath, 1799]. Reprint of Article XVI, Volume IX, of the *Transactions of the Bath and West of England Society*.

N° 24 **24**

Bath June 30th 1792

My dear Sir

A journey to London on urgent business together with a variety of dispatches on sundry occasions have till this moment so completely occupied my whole time that I have not had even a chance of answering your former letter till lo! a 2nd has just arrived w^h involves a question of no small moment. To answer this with propriety and in proportion to its importance I must confess myself more at a loss than on my former occasion. Your predilection for anatomy I concluded had given you a decided preference for surgery, to w^h however it now appears that you have a dislike, and propose to content yourself with [the] humble department of pharmacy for w^h you have contracted a strong partiality. Your mother's kind wish and approbation for your continuing another year at Edin^r can never be sufficiently acknowledged, an indulgence w^h claims your warmest thanks, your warmest gratitude. After this, y^r own feelings, y^r own inclination guided by y^r own discretion will determine y^r choice better than any other person can determine for you. However as you seem anxious to hear my opinion, I will briefly [word missing?] my sentiments, tho' in a matter of such moment, I cannot pretend to advise. Should you fix in Bristol or some great city y^r original plan of surgery and midwifery might be sufficient alone. If in a country town, pharmacy seems a necess^y appendage to the other two, and a sine qua non, if you wholly decline surgery. But s^{hd} surgery after all be y^{r} chief branch, half a year in Lond^{n} either this or the next winter might be sufficient for an anatomical course and dissections, with occasional visits to some of the London hospitals. But to enter regul^{y} at any of the great hospitals it will cost you at least 20 ^{Gs}, and above double the sum as surg^{y} pupil.[1] As to the more humble station of an apothecary, many people wou'd think you have already done that department, not considering that in this country the apoth^{y} is literally the physician, the all in all in the widely diversified field of physic. The great doctor in the big wig is indeed as a matter of form, and now and then to lend a hand at a dead lift, occasionally had recourse to. But the apoth^{ys} mortar sounds aloud, and his introduction to practice is more smooth, easy and expeditious—his journeys are regularly expected; and the score for d^{fts} and boluses steals silently on long after the great D^{r} is dismissed. Midwifery is a key by w^{h} he gains admission to the ladies' hearts as well as their nurses—a child or 2 are unwell, or may be by and by—and who so fit to take care of them as the dear tender-hearted man who brought them into y^{e} world, or was perhaps instrumental towards their very existence? You have the theory of midwifery, only want a little more practical knowledge, and then with a snug well-stored shop, value 50$^{£}$, with a golden label over the door—J.W., Apoth^{y} and Accoucheur—you may start & boldly declare—"Opiferque per orbem dicor."[2] When in town, at a meeting of the Royal Society I was accosted by Dr Gregory[3] who of his own accord spoke of you what I was very willing to hear, but need not repeat, as all acc^{ts} agree that you are driving on Jehu[4] like, and "that y^{r} progress keeps pace with y^{r} diligence." Now since the height of y^{r} ambition is to be an apoth^{y}, that is a retailer of drugs, an administerer of clysters and carrier out of gallipots, as the name of y^{r} brethren plainly implies—A-pot-he-carries, I flatter myself that in time you may be qualified for this high calling. One supposition more, and I have done. Suppose Apollo the God of Physic, tho' once only a collector of herbs or rather strolling apoth^{y} sh^{d} after all whisper in y^{r} ear—"Why all this anxious preparation, this long toil and study to sit down an understrapper at last? Why sit down at ye foot of ye hill of science with powers sufficient to gain the summit? and when one winter more will conduct you to the 'primis in medicina honoribus'[5] and entitle you to an upper seat in my temple? But then you must wait with patience till the blossoms w^{h} hang over my shrine ripen into fruit, and learn to live on aethereal air as many of my votaries are obliged to do 2 or 3 seasons before they are admitted to pluck the 'aureum pomum'[6]"—If you listen to these suggestions, and can afford to wait, you'll stay where you are and push on with y^{r} wonted alacrity, only add a course of theory of medicine and devoting ye time allotted for English, to Latin, read^{g} Celsus[7] and van Swieten. Before you finally determine, reconsider ye matter well. Consult y^{r} mother and y^{r} relations etc. The pros and cons are now before you "Nullum numen abest si sit Prudentia."[8] That you may determine wisely is the ardent wish of Dr Sir y^{rs}

A. Fothergill

P.S. My best respects to Drs Duncan, Gregory and others who kindly countenance you and to whose able admonitions I recommend you and to show all possible attention to 'em.
P.S. July 15 This lett^{r} was ready a fortnight ago as the date expresses, but being sent to Dr Hawes, who is an able judge, for his opinion w^{h} I now find coincides with my own. But instead of forwarding ye lett^{r} to you as desired, he forgets, and sends it back here this day from whence it is now dispatched. Purposes will happen!

[1] See letter **16**, note 3.

[2] "And I am called throughout the world the aid-bringer" Apollo, the god of medicine, is the speaker. Ovid, *Metamorphoses*, 1.521.

[3] James Gregory, since 1790 the professor of the practice of medicine in the university of Edinburgh.

[4] A coachman, especially one who drives at a rattling pace. "The watchman told, saying . . . The driving is like the driving of Jehu the son of Nimshi; for he driveth furiously". 2 Kings ix, 20.

[5] "Foremost honours in medicine".

[6] "The golden apple".

[7] One of the many editions of A. Cornelius Celsus (*fl.* 1st century AD), *De medicina libri octo*, called the "Cicero medicorum" for the elegance of his Latin.

[8] "No deity is absent, if there be prudence". Juvenal, *Satires*, 10.365. See also letter **19**.

N° 26 **25**

Bath 8^ber [October] 6th 1792

Your very obliging letter, my dear sir, is just arrived, and tho' I am very busy, I cannot omit answering it immediately, and am glad opportunity offers of a safe conveyance to Newcastle where this letter will be expedited by the post. I am truly concerned to hear of your indisposition which is evidently of the hypocond^l kind and plainly brought on by too intense application and the want of due exercise and amusement. If I am right in my conjecture as to the cause, the cure I hope will not be difficult. But then you must resolutely observe ye following rules, for these blue devils must absolutely be brushed off or they will take possession of you and render you a moping useless being. But remember you are born to nobler ends, therefore banish spleen—banish melancholy. Allow yourself 2 hours for brisk exercise every day, whether in fencing, dancing or riding a rough-trotting horse, which last is the best because ye exercise is in the open air. Devote 2 or 3 evenings in a week to music or convivial meetings, but exclude all intemperance. Never study close immediately after a full meal. When the languor and depression are very great take a glass of Julep c[um] Camph[or] with a spoonful of Vin Croci[1] and Tinct: Cort Huxh:[2] Of nights restless—Syr [?]h.s.[3] By the above method I hope you'll soon regain your wonted health and vivacity. But you must not think ye time lost that is to be thus devoted to exercise. Remember health is too important to be sacrificed to books and solitude. I am pleased to hear that your associates are selected from amongst the most respectable students—the sons of the professors. Those that are communicative and of good morals merit your attention, and their friendship deserves to be cultivated. As to y^r destination, I have set before you the pros and cons—you and y^r friends must determine. From what I have stated you'll easily gather my opinion and also that of Dr Hawes, and we shall both at pleasure ruminate on y^r pres^t proposal w^h is not without its objections. What says your mother, brothers, etc? What in short wou'd be y^r own choice? I hoped by this time you had consulted them and determined the question. For this ought to determine your ensuing course of studies. But whatever be y^r destination, remember to take care of y^r health and not forfeit it to y^r passion for books. For that wou'd be bad policy and wou'd also frustrate every purpose. You attempted too much last y^r—you must be more discreet this season. If you attend theory of medicine, anat^y and clinical lectures—quite enough. Materia medica you may collect from authors. If you can get elected at Med^l Soc^y you must not be balked for a little sum[4]—so enter if you can—and let me know if cash is likely to run too short to make both ends meet before the conclusion of the lectures. Beware of purchasing many books the carriage of w[h] you'll find a weighty additional expense at last. Your course of reading is good, but you need not be so anxious about the Latin, the exam[n5]—or the space before practice becomes in some degree productive. Excuse haste and believe me my worthy youth y[rs]

assuredly
A. Fothergill

P.S. The papers lately announced the fatal hydrophobia at Edin[r] of w[h] I shall be glad to hear the particulars. Various avocations retard my essay on that subject.[6] In June I accidentally fell in with Professor Gregory at the Royal Society tho' I did not know him at that instant nor till he was gone.[7] Please to remember me to him and also to Professor Monro.[8] The Edin[r] new Pharmc[a] will I suppose appear 'ere long.[9] Adieu!

1 Saffron wine.
2 Tinct Cort Huxh refers to Huxham's compound tincture of bark (cinchona). Fothergill prescribed two drachms in Apothecary signs.
3 Refers to six drachms (in Apothecary signs) of a syrup to be taken at bedtime: h.s.—hora somni. The syrup's name is indecipherable but the context suggests Syrupus e Meconio. This opiate was prepared from poppy heads.
4 See letter **20**, note 2.
5 That is the MD examination.
6 See letter **23**, note 11.
7 This is extremely odd, since in June (letter **24**) Fothergill reported speaking to Gregory at the Royal Society.
8 Alexander Monro, *secundus*.
9 Presumably, *Pharmacopoeia collegii regii medicorum Edinburgensis*, Edinburgh, Bell & Bradfute, 1792.

N[o] 25 **26**

Bath Nov: 22nd 1792

Dr Sir

Having with some difficulty procured this frank, time I fear will hardly permit me to fill it much less supply an enclosure expatiating on the different topics of y[r] last letter. My last of the preceding week left with D[r] Hawes (with a request that he would fill up the vacant space with a postscript), I hope you have received, w[h] will leave but little to add at present. For tho' friends may state their opinion in the most full and disinterested manner respecting y[r] destination, it must still rest with you and y[r] relations ultimately to determine. In the present lottery of medical affairs there is no possibility of insuring success—the most eligible and the most promising plan sometimes fails, while a random hit succeeds, and leads on to fortune and distinction. For my own part I have no very high opinion of those lucky hits w[h] may or may not occur independent of real merit. An ingenuous mind must shrink back abashed on receiving honours etc., emoluments it is conscious of being in no wise entitled to. Let it be your study to frame your own fortune on the basis of a good education, and to depend more on prudence and propriety of conduct than on fortunate contingencies, or even the recommendation of friends. In a word, I wish you to become as much as possible (whatever y^r lot may be) independent of fortune, and what Horace pronounces concerning the man of virtue and integrity "Totus teres atque rotundus."[1] Y^r case of hydrophobia appears to be very accurately and circumstantially delineated whether drawn from hospital reports or y^r own immediate observation. In the 1st stage it partook more of febrile diathesis than is, I believe common, and yet the phenomena after death testified no evident marks of inflammation. Whether the pain etc. extending along the arm marked out absorption or only nervous irritation does not appear—had reddish lines along the lymphatics from the wound, attended with soreness and tenderness of the axillary gland, been observed, it wou'd have afforded a strong presumptive proof of the virus being absorbed. The clinical professor and sev^l students wou'd doubtless have [had] an eye to this and noted every phenomenon in his lecture. The other symptoms and fatal termination confirm what has been too often observed in similar cases. The 3rd day from the commencement of the dread of liquids was accordingly the fatal period. But ye 1st stage afforded more openings for the use of vigorous measures than common, but despair of success seems in this and some other cases to have prevented the physician from availing himself of them till it was too late! Perhaps some new thesis on that subject may be obtained. My M.S.[on hydrophobia] remains dormant till Dr Lettsom's translation of an American thesis with notes appears,[2] w^h may perhaps surpass my observations. Mr Dawson's compt^s. I have only room to add the best wishes of Dear Sir,

y^rs assuredly A. Fothergill

[1] "Whole, smooth, and well-rounded". Horace, *Satires*, 2.7.86.

[2] James Mease (1771–1846), *An essay on the disease produced by the bite of a mad dog, or other rabid animal. . . . With a preface and appendix by J. C. Lettsom*, London, C. Dilly, 1793.

N° 27 **27**

Bath Decr 24/92

Your excellent letter, my Dear Sir, addressed to Dr Hawes containing many warm expressions of gratitude which do credit both to the head and heart of the writer has just now been communicated to me. As Dr Hawes may be too busy to send an immediate reply, I am sit down (tho' by no means at leisure) to answer it in his part as well as my own, and am happy to have engaged in y^r interest so warm and steady a friend as Dr Hawes. I hope you received my last wherein I expressed a wish that he cou'd be elected an Hon^y Member of the Royal Med^l Soc^y of Edin^r and cou'd now wish that it cou'd be brought about by y^r means, as it would attach him still more closely to y^r interest, and I know wou'd be highly grateful to him, and add to his éclat as he is about to publish a vol. addressed to the King as Patron of the Humane Society.[1] His modesty will not permit him to speak out for himself, and his professional character stands already too high to solicit it. So that by elect^g him the Soc^y wou'd receive as well as confer honour. Therefore please to make strict inquiry as to the present rules respect^g the elect^n of hon^y members—whether a person must have studied at Edin^r? been an ordinary member a certain time? whether a young member can propose him? whether elected by ballot? and what majority requires it? If the 2 first circumstances are essential he has no chance and the matter drops. In that case write him an account of the rules without hinting my present interposition in his favour, and that as soon as you can, but without seeming to write expressly on that topic. I am hearty glad of your own introduction into the Society, and if you can find means to carry his elect^{n} by interest with senior members I know you'll not be wanting in zeal or assiduity. But shou'd he be proposed and rejected, I trust it will never reach his ears. I am much pleased and so is Dr Hawes to hear you have at length formed a resolution of becoming a candidate for a D^{rs} degree tho' it was too delicate a point for us to urge, or even persuade you to without the entire concurrence of yourself and friends. I trust that they nor you will ever see cause to repent it. You'll do well, however, to consider this may be accomplished in 2 years, the term allowed by ye College, as well as in 3 ^{yrs}.[2] If so why add the heavy expense of an additional year? If you cannot equip yourself in 2 years as well as many others do in 3 or even 4 years I have made a wrong estimate of y^{r} abilities and y^{r} assiduity. Not that I mean you shou'd kill yourself by overstudy in order to reach your imagined acme of perfection by running against time. No, take care of your health first; secondly of y^{r} study and thirdly of your purse, or rather your poor mother's. So as the Dutch express it, I must leave this ad referendum. The late cautions and instructions I suggested have, I hope, not been thrown away as to any of these important points, and as you are silent as to bodily complaints I flatter myself your health is tolerably reestablished. I approve much of the plan of study you are now engaged in: anatomy, clinical lectures and clinical practice, van Swieten, with the result of fatal diseases as illustrated by Morgagni. Your time, I am convinced, cannot admit of long letters, much less encountering any essay except your future thesis, and this you should lose no time in bringing forward unless you determine not to graduate next summer. You shou'd habituate yourself to speak and write in Latin as the College, I fear, will not cordially allow of an exam^{n} in English as the Dublin College has wisely done. Read van Swieten much and also Celsus, they will give you easy and elegant diction. Turn English into Latin and Latin into English, and if there be any Latin book on the anim^{l} oeconomy in [the] form of dialogue, strive to get it. If not, I may perhaps supply the defect by a short manuscript previous to y^{r} examinations.[3] Remember the sooner you get on the toga medica, the sooner you will begin to reap the fruits of it, and the more time you will have to see practice in London and reconnoitre the country for a vacancy. I shall not expect to hear from you till you have made up y^{r} mind on this matter. My respects to y^{r} kind preceptors and friends, and believe me, my Dr Sir, much yours A. Fothergill

N.B. Blacker ink and a rounder hand will add to the pleasure of reading your letters not a little

N.B. Mr Dawson's respects

[1] Presumably, William Hawes, *Modes of treatment for the recovery of drowned persons*, 1793.

[2] Fothergill was mistaken, see Introduction, p. xx.

[3] Fothergill does seem to have supplied such a catechism, which was subsequently lost. See letters **32**, **42**, and **46**.

N° 75 **28**

Bath Feb 1st 1793

Dr Madam,[1]

Your son having with yr consent and that of his relations and friends determined to graduate at Edinr he wrote to me some time ago that he proposed to continue his stay at the university and equip himself for a Drs degree against the summer 1794. Knowing his course of preparatory studies his diligence and abilities, I strongly advised him to finish at Edinr the ensuing summer 1793 by wh both time and expense wou'd be saved, but in his letter just now arrived, he assures me that by a new regulation in the College since my time, it now requires instead of two, three years to obtain a Drs degree.[2] A circumstance unknown to me and wh will, necessarily, greatly enhance the expense. By strict oeconomy however and diligence wh I have every reason to believe regulates his whole conduct, I hope in due time he will still surmount this and every other difficulty and amply repay the debt of gratitude due to an indulgent mother. He has, I make no doubt, informed you that in compliance with his request I lent him Octr 14 1791 ten pounds, the receipt of wh he acknowledges in a subsequent lettr. At present I find he is in great want of a further remittance. If you cannot spare him 10£, I will, if you desire it, endeavour to procure it, and send him a bank bill of that amount per post as before. But as life is uncertain and accidents may happen, it is but reasonable that I shd have security fm you or yr promissory note, on a stamp, in some such form as the following, wh as soon as I receive, I will take care no time is lost in procuring and forwarding the money to yr son, and in the interim remain with best wishes, Dr Madam

your very humble servant
A. Fothergill

I promise to pay Dr Anthony Fothergill on order twenty pounds for cash advanced to my son Mr John [*sic*] Woodforde student of physic at Edinr at different times viz. Octr 14th 1791 and Feb__1793 as witness my hand £ 20
P.S. Perhaps you may rather choose to supply him with the present sum yourself and then your note to me will be only £10.

[1] This letter, to Woodforde's mother, seems to confirm the suggestion that the Woodfordes were unknown to the transcriber, since James is referred to as John.
[2] See Introduction, p. xx.

N° 28 **29**

Bath Feby: 10th 1793

Dear Sir,

I am truly concerned to hear that by some late regulation of the College, candidates cannot now be received for graduation under 3 years, When I fully expected the affair would be completed the ensuing summer! If ever this hard law is dispensed with, I hope it still may [be] in your favour, as it cannot be denied that pupils who come well prepared and to genius add indefatigable assiduity, will make greater progress in 2 years than others without these qualifications usually do in 3 years. If this indulgence cannot be obtained a trip to Leyden this summ^r may finish the business without another year at Edin^r [which] must inevitably add greatly to your expense, and it remains for y^r consideration, and that of y^r relations whether you will submit to it, or graduate this sum^r at some other University or finally contract y^r plan to the humble station of surgeon and apothecary as proposed originally till you can in some measure reimburse yourself. In the interim, oeconomy, rigid oeconomy will, as you observe, be absolutely necessary. Soon after your letter arrived, I wrote to y^r mother on this unexpected dilemma, and mentioned your necessity as to a remittance, offering that if it was not quite convenient to her to send you a £10 bill, I wou'd, on her dropping a line with her promissory note on a stamp for the whole advanced on your acc^t, as wou'd be but reasonable considering the extreme uncertainty of life. Having waited her answer till this moment, I fully conclude she had or will soon send you the remittance herself. This is fortunate, for a friend just now has requested me to join him in the purchase of some ground rents—to w^h I have agreed and the purchase money will, I find, not only require all my present cash, but, even the loan of a moderate sum for which I must pay 5 per cent. In case your remittance sh^d not be speedy the enclosed commission from Mr Dawson, may perhaps put a little cash in your hands for the present and you can request your mother to repay him the like sum here. I am pleased to hear of your progress and see your visible improvement in the epistolary way. With a few general rules from your Latin master you may now dispense with his attendance and spend 1 hour as usual on that language, in prose rather than verse unless you had more time. As soon as the ballot is over write directly to Dr Hawes the result, meanwhile use every effort to gain votes and ensure success. He knows that his name has been proposed. May he receive good tidings and may you have the pleasure of communicating them in the sincere wish of Dr Sir, yours sincerely

A. Fothergill

P.S. My best respects to Dr Gregory, and your other preceptors who distinguish you by their kindness and attention. N.B. I forward this under cover to Lond^n w^h will lighten postage

N° 29 **30**

Bath March 10th 1793

Dear Sir,

Tho' very busy, I think it necessary to answer your letter just arrived, immediately. Hitherto, as you well know, I have anxiously avoided dictating, or even advising as to your future destination. This, I repeatedly desired you to determine yourself at leisure after due deliberation with your relations. Having at length declared your resolution for graduation, the term of w^{h} it seems is altered from 2 to 3 y^{rs} w^{h} will of course make near 100$^{£}$ difference in the expense. I hinted to your friends that if the expense cou'd not be complied with, there was but this alternative, either to relinquish the plan, or to graduate at Leyden this summer, not that it wou'd be more eligible, and even reputable to graduate at Edin^{r}. Many, it is true, for similar prudential reasons go over to Leyden and if a degree can be had there (as I presume it may after 2 y^{r}. study at Edin^{r}, of wch however you can easily satisfy yourself from the students as to the laws of that university) you can then soon determine with your relations accordingly. For I neither can, nor dare venture to advise. Holland at present is agitated by warlike alarms but the contest is likely to be soon over, and I have not heard that medical affairs at Leyden are even at this time interrupted. This university is doubtless held in a more reputable point of view than any Scotch seminary, Edin^{r} excepted. Had you resolved to sit down a mere apoth^{y},1 year at Edin^{r} wou'd have been sufficient and more than falls to the lot of the generality of pharmacopolists according to the present system of education. To complete the education of a phys^{n} he sh^{d} have an independence of 100 or $^{£}$150 per annum to set out with, but as you entered well prepared it is but fair to reckon you have at least a year start of y^{r} competitors who entered mere novices at the time you went to Edin^{r} and consequently that your 2nd year is at least equal to their 3rd year which qualifies you to graduate this summ^{r}. But when a physician has taken his degree you'll recollect what I have formerly observed, that much time, patience and assiduity are still necessary to introduce him by slow degrees into medical practice and that the present rage for educating young men as physicians has so considerably overstocked the profession in every eligible station as to render their introduction and progress still more difficult. Unless the rules of the Leyden college require that the candidate shou'd enter the classes there previous to graduation, I should think it wholly unnecessary. The thesis is, I believe, always printed at Leyden. The epilepsy is by no means a very frequent disease, or so popular as many others you'll have to encounter in practice such as smallpox inoculation, rhum^{m}, phthysis pulmonalis, catarrh, angina, typhus etc. Not but that every tyro sh^{d} choose his own subject. It will be necessary to converse in Latin either with the pupils or a Latinist to acquire facility in answering the questions at the different examinations. A thesis of 20 or 30 pages may be written in English and translated, and lastly corrected by a Latinist.[1] If so able a practit^{r} as Dr Pearson[2] has been rejected it is an unfavorable omen for Dr Hawes, tho' of much longer standing. But the dye is cast, and by this time his fate determined. Sorry—I shall be extremely sorry if it has gone against him. If so he must be told it in the most gentle and soothing manner. I regret young Percival's death, the son of my venerable correspondent and contempor^{y}, Dr Percival.[3] Also the other youth, especially if son of some of my old friends from Dublin. None of the theses of last summer have arrived at Bath, only the titles, some of which appear interesting, particularly on submersion, poisons,[4] etc. If you determine for Leyden, the time and every particular requisite thereto sh^{d} be well learnt at Edin^{r}, and no time lost in the preparative requisites. If on the other hand y^{r} friends consent to another year at Edin^{r}, your Leyden journey will be spared. Whatever may be their determination you have the best wishes of, Dr Sir, y^{rs} sincerely

A. Fothergill

[1] The MD examination was conducted in Latin. The student was first examined orally at the home of one of the professors. The student then submitted his thesis, following which he was examined by two

professors in the presence of the faculty. He then had to give a written explanation of two Hippocratic aphorisms and then a written commentary on two cases, which had to be defended orally. See Christopher Lawrence, 'Medicine as culture: Edinburgh and the Scottish Enlightenment', University of London, PhD thesis, 1984, pp. 197–200.

[2] I.e. rejected for honorary membership of the RMS. Possibly, George Pearson (1751–1828), MD (Edinburgh 1773), FRS, physician and chemist; or Richard Pearson (1765–1836), MD (Edinburgh 1786), physician; or John Pearson (1758–1826), FRS, surgeon, member of the RMS in 1820.

[3] Thomas Percival, MD (Leyden 1765), FRS, physician and founding member of the Manchester Literary and Philosophical Society (1781). James Percival, his son, died in 1793 while finishing his medical studies in Edinburgh. See letter from 'Dr. Percival to Dr. Haygarth', Manchester, 1793, in *Memoirs of the life and writings of Thomas Percival MD*, London, Richard Cruttwell for J. Johnson, 1807, pp. clxxvii-clxxix, cclv-cclvi.

[4] Edinburgh MD theses for 1792 included Jacobus Davidson, *De vita submersorum resucitanda*. There was no thesis on poisons.

N° 30 **31**

Bath June 16 1793

About a fortnight ago, my Dear Sir, I was favored with your obliging letter which various engagements have obliged me to postpone answering till now. It is with peculiar satisfaction that I find your mother has given her free consent to your continuing at Edin^r another year, for w^h act of maternal affection and indulgence she merits all the thanks and all the gratitude that filial duty and obedience can bestow and I flatter myself that her well timed liberality will in the end be amply repaid, and that neither she nor you will have cause to repent of the additional time and expense which the change in y^r destination necessarily requires. As this favour was rather to be hoped for than expected I need not add that it will be incumbent upon you to employ it to the utmost advantage, and that with a strict eye to oeconomy. Tho' it is true you might, this summer, [have] passed muster with as good a grace as some of longer standing yet the consciousness of having completed your education in a more ample manner must add greatly to y^r own satisfaction when you sit down to practice. Having moreover fulfilled the laws of the 1st medical school in Europe will give additional éclat to your first setting out, on w^h so much often depends. I am pleased to hear that your progress keeps pace with y^r diligence and application, and that the rugged brow of science begins to wear a more smooth and engaging aspect. This will continue to brighten as you advance, but think not that you are nearly arrived at the summit. For at that moment you'll find, as Pope elegantly expresses it:

"Hills peep o'er hills, and Alps on Alps arise!"[1]

Tho' much is done, much you'll find still remains to be executed, for science is boundless "Qui studet optatam cursu contingere metam/ multa tulit fecitque puer."—Horace[2]

I fear you still [have] too many irons in the fire and must request you not to waste time on things trifling or indifferent, for tho' you have 1 year before you, it will quickly slide away. Spend not too much time on the papers for the societies, nor on botany beyond the 1st lines of the Linnean system much less on miscellan^s correspondence. You say after ye elapse of 3 months, instead of lapse. Time elapses, but the substantive is lapse. However this is only a lapsus calami[3] and the only lapse I have met with in your late letters. D^r

Hawes and I are both convinced that his want of success was not owing to any want of exertion on your part. He bears it with philosophy and has promised me to write to you (as is utmost due) a grateful letter, and also hints about your thesis but I think the choice must be left to yourself. I see no objection to typhus, a beaten track will require less time and trouble than to cut a new road thro' a trackless forest. Haller's Methodus Studii Medici[4] will supply a list of practical authors on malig[t] fevers—van Swieten and Hoffman will afford matter to be improved on by Cullen and late writers—also Theses de Typho in Smellie and Webster's collection.[5] From what I have said you stand higher with D[r] Hawes than ever, and so far from being offended we both are sensible of y[r] services, and kind intention. Amidst the fashionable failures are 2 of the Bath banks. By one of w[h] I shall sustain a very heavy loss. But I feel more sensibly for many of my fellow citizens who have lost their all!!! When you have once fixed on a subject for a thesis, begin without delay. Take time by the forelock for behind he is quite bald—"Nullus dies sine linea."[6] My respects to your preceptors. Consult them when difficulties occur, and go on with alacrity. Collect materials from the best sources, leave blank leaf and open lines for corrections, and now my D[r] Sir, Vale! et cave ut valeas![7]

A. Fothergill

[1] Alexander Pope (1688–1744), *An essay on criticism*, 1. 232.

[2] "He who strains to attain the longed-for goal on the race-course has endured and done much while still a boy". Horace, *Art of poetry*, 412–13.

[3] Slip of the pen.

[4] Presumably, Hermann Boerhaave, *Methodus studii medici. Emaculata & accessionibus locupletata ab Alberto ab Haller*, 2 vols., Amsterdam, J. a Wetstein, 1751.

[5] William Smellie (1740–1795), *Thesaurus medicus: sive disputationum in Academia Edinensi ad rem medicam pertinentium . . . delectus*, 4 vols., Edinburgh, Typis Academicus, 1778–85; and Charles Webster (1750–1795), *Medicinæ praxeos systema ex academia Edinburgenae disputationibus praecipue inauguralibus depromptum*, 3 vols., Edinburgh, J. Bell & R. Murray for W. Gordon and R. Murray, 1781.

[6] "No day without a line". Proverb mentioned in Pliny, *Historia naturalis*, 35, 84. I.e., no day without some work on one's art, supposed originally to describe how the Greek painter Apelles went to work.

[7] "Farewell! and take care you keep well". Not attributable. See also letters **32**, **33**, **82**, and **84**.

N[o] 31 **32**

Bath Oct[r] 10th 1793

Before me, Dear Sir, is your affectionate letter, and am happy to hear that y[r] health and spirits enable you to pursue your studies with y[r] wonted alacrity and w[h] in time will I hope be crowned with academical honours. Tho' I have little to add to the admonitions already offered, I cannot let slip this opportunity of throwing off a few hasty lines by M[r] B. D[awson's] packet w[h] is ready, and only waits for this. But what I think will be of much greater importance and enable you to approach the dread tribunal (before which you must 'ere long appear) with a more firm step and more steady countenance I enclose for y[r] careful perusal a few M.S. of preparatory exercises ready cut and dry w[h] you may soon make yourself master of and have at your fingers ends ready to be played off on the day you are attacked. For my wish is that you may appear unabashed before the Solemn Court of

Inquisition serena fronte,[1] and answer their interrogatories ore rotundo.[2] If you think the list not sufficy ample, your own ingenuity and knowledge of the trim of the College may suggest to you a few more, together with the responses according to the theory of the times by way of appendix. Thus armed at all points you may like the hedgehog roll yourself up snug, and bid defiance to all their artillery, and perhaps even wound some of your less powerful assailants in the encounter. 40 candidates for next session!!![3] You my worthy élève amongst this number must enter the lists, and must expect to meet with some very able competitors, but will I trust be found not the last in the race, nor the least deserving the laurel wreath.

As to yr subject, tho' I hinted what I thought ineligible, I wou'd not direct what you shou'd fix on but left it to your choice. For one drowned person you will in practice meet with at least a dozen cases of typhus. As your thesis on that is nearly finished, suppose you shew both in confidence to Drs D[uncan] or G[regory] and request their candid opinion; which they think most advisable or best adapted to yr present views, or future prospects. The one omitted, if found valuable, may still appear on some future occasion if necessary.

Your chief bent this winter must be towards the practice. This with clinl lects, the Infiry and perusal of suitable practl writers, finishing and retouching yr thesis, will find you very full employment. Therefore lose not time in writg any lettrs that can be omitted. But, Perge et respice finem.[4] If you can imitate the concise neat style of Celsus or even the easy perspicuous one of van Swieten which, tho' less elegant and less Roman, is perhaps much more intelligible and therefore more useful, you need not a better model. But the translation of yr thesis will cost you more labour than you are aware of, therefore the sooner you get thro' it ye better as it will need twice polishing. Compare ye rates of paper and printing at different presses, you'll want but a few copies on fine paper and must study oeconomy, not vie with ye extravagant sons of fortune. Yr letters are easy, natural and well expressed but require a microscopic eye, as this does at present, wh is a fault tho' not of great magnitude. Now my, Dr Sir, adieu!

Vale! and cave ut valeas![5]

A. Fothergill

[1] "With untroubled brow". Not attributable.

[2] "With well-rounded diction". Horace, *Art of poetry*, 323.

[3] There were actually 29 graduates in 1794. See *List of graduates in medicine in the University of Edinburgh*, Edinburgh, Neill & Company, 1867, p. 25.

[4] "Go ahead and have regard to the end". Not attributable.

[5] "Farewell! and take care you keep well". See also letters **31**, **33**, **82**, and **84**.

N° 32 **33**

Bath New Year's Day 1794

My dear Sir,

Tho' pressed for time beyond measure and obliged to postpone answering all letters unless on urgent business, yet I cannot let this day slip without felicitating you on your late hair breadth escape and on your entering on a new year. Most sincerely do I rejoice that you are still in the land of the living and that your progress towards perfect recovery is so promising. Much is due to your kind preceptors for their humane attention and also to the worthy family with whom you lodge. Amidst strangers and remote from your relations, how deplorable must your situation have been had it not been for the friendly aid of these good Samaritans! Having thus escaped shipwreck it is hoped you will not endanger your health and life again by embarking too suddenly, or before you have recovered sufficient firmness—"non bene ripæ / creditur. Ipse aries etiam nunc vellera siccat."[1]

A relapse remember, is sometimes worse than the original disease. But your worthy physic^{s} I make no doubt have given you every necess^{y} caution on this head. The anxiety we lately felt on your account can only be equaled by the joy we now experience. I cannot help adding my hearty approbation of the classes you propose to attend previous to your examinations. Your having your thesis in such forwardness was a happy circumstance, and its having passed in form of a case the Med^{l} Soc^{y} with applause will enable you to retouch it where weak, or correct exceptionable or doubtful passages.[2] Van Swieten was always a great favorite and by consulting him you'll find a fund of useful facts, and from his simplicity and perspicuity improve your Latinity. Haller's Elementa Physiologiae 8 tom.[3] must be also considered, tho' too voluminous to be read thro' at this time. The Edin^{r} Encyclopedia[4] will deserve to be dipped into on certain points, and also the English Cyclopedia.[5] I am glad the M.S. reached you safe and shall be much pleased if it proves useful, as a preparatory to your approaching trial and enable you to appear

"Totus teres atque rotundus." [6]

For other particulars medical, oeconomical or prudential, I refer you to my former letters, and now I must hastily conclude with my best wishes for your health and success and y^{t} you may live to see many happy new years

Dear Sir vale! et cave ut valeas![7]

A. Fothergill

[1] "There is no trusting the river bank. The ram himself is still drying his fleece". Virgil, *Eclogues*, 3.94–5.
[2] See Introduction, p. xxi.
[3] Von Haller, *Elementa physiologiae*, see letter **6**, note 2.
[4] *Encyclopedia Britannica* perhaps. See letter **23**, note 10.
[5] Possibly E. Chambers, *Cyclopaedia; or an universal dictionary of arts and sciences*, 2 vols., London, James & John Knapton, 1728. Another edition, 5 vols., J. F. and C. Rivington, 1791, 1779–89.
[6] "Whole, smooth and well-rounded". Horace, *Satires*, 2.7.86. See also letter **26**.
[7] "Farewell! and take care you keep well". See also letters **31**, **32**, **82**, and **84**.

N° 33 **34**

Bath April 10th 1794

Your obliging letter, my Dear Sir, arrived about 5 days ago and brought me the welcome tidings of your health being reestablished—a mercy w^{h} claims the most profound tribute of gratitude, adoration and praise to that Being who overrules all events, and "whose mercy is over all his works"!!! Such a signal deliverance, and at such an important period in y[r] life ought to make such an impression on your mind as never to be obliterated! The eldest son of my worthy friend D[r] Lettsom[1] is, I understand, prosecuting his med[l] studies at Edin[r]. A fine promising youth with whom you should be acquainted. The beadle or porter of y[e] College will inform you where he lodges. Tell him, at my request, you take the liberty to wait on him, and to inquire if you can render him any acceptable service from your previous acquaintance in the place, and assure him of my best wishes for his success. Let this be your introduction. If my last afforded you some consolation when just beginning to emerge from a most dangerous illness, I trust this will tend to fortify you against that fear and trepidation w[h] usually precedes the first examination. You can but be remanded to y[r] studies, so you know the worst that can happen and may still do for a country a pot he carry—the summit of your early ambition. And tho' of 30 candidates[2] you should be the only one doomed to wield the pestle, why never mind it, since the present Duke of Orleans of blood royal and born to an estate of more than £50,000 per annum is content to be usher to a country school master, while his royal relation, the heir apparent, is confined to a loathsome prison!

Let us suppose you for a moment, in a state of arrest and summonsed to take your trial before the revolutionary tribunal with Danton and other conspirators, why still you wou'd have this consolation, that you cou'd but lose your head, and that amongst orators and legislators, the very best of company. Fortunately however you are not in a state of arrest, and have not to face a tribunal whose judges are your enemies, or a corrupt jury bent on your destination but a tribunal distinguished for mildness and candor whose judges are your preceptors, y[r] friends, your well-wishers, indulgent to venial errors, and encouragers of modest merit, who know how to make allowance for little slips which may arise from timidity, or want of presence of mind after such a severe illness, all of which, if you see necessity, you may in a short preface avail yourself. Banish then from this moment all childish fears, reperuse the letter of the 20th.[3] Drink a bumper of wine (for I hear you are become a complete wine bibber) and then march up to the tribunal serena fronte.[4] Strike out of your thesis every superfluous word which only weakens y[r] language. Aim at the conciseness of Celsus, and reduce, if possible, your 40 to 30 pages. Unfold the principles in a masterly outline, and leave somewhat to the discernment of the reader to fill up. Remember you address not the vulgar but the erudite, ready to anticipate your argumentation. Avoid, above all things, every unnecessary expense. Y[r] friends promised to supply the needful, but rely on your strict oeconomy, and that you will not engage in any unnecess[y] tour in things fit only for the affluent. Your Latinity depends more on conversing and your own industry than on a teacher. The books you read are very proper, to w[h] add Celsus for the sake of his language. Avoid writing letters till the whole be over, your time is doubly precious, and I can easily conceive what is passing. Collect theses, and watch every new improvement but tarry not longer than necessary

With best wishes for your happy deliverance
I am Dear Sir, yours assuredly

A. Fothergill

My respects to any who may inquire after me.

[1] John Coakley Lettsom's son, John Miers Lettsom (1771–1800).
[2] See letter **32**, note 3.
[3] If this refers to one of Fothergill's letters, it is missing, along, probably, with many others.
[4] "With untroubled brow". See also letter **32**.

No 34 **35**

Bath May 28th 1794

Dear Sir,

Your obliging letter which arrived here 3 days brings me the welcome news of yr having passed the private ordeal[1] with much credit. This I persuade myself affords a happy omen that yr public examination will be performed with no less éclat. In the interim I need not exhort you to lose no time in making all necessary preparation, in anticipating the questions and responses, and guarding yr Latinity from vulgarisms & false concord. For it demands no small presence of mind to speak a dead language correctly, and make the responses pointedly in public before such an august assembly of medical and literary critics. It may not be amiss to prepare yr first response with a short apology for any lapsus linguæ that may possibly escape you from the awe wh the appearing before such a learned assembly must naturally inspire. On very doubtful or intricate points it is fair to hesitate a little and better to give modest than a pert reply or peremptory—as ut mihi videtur[2]—or cum pace eruditissimi professoris[3]—or ea qua par est deferentia doctissimo præceptori.[4] Let your M.S. be written fair and not too small, and correct the press yourself with great care submitting the punctuation to the composition. A multiplicity of margin[l] or other notes increase the trouble and expense of printing, and also look pedantic and are becoming unfashionable. Paper and printing being very dear, I should think 200 copies quite sufficient, and will require you not to be too prodigal in the distribution, saying you have several friends in England to whom copies will be indispensable. Perhaps a dozen or 2 should be on fine paper, but no occasion for marbled covers. But Mr Mcaulay must know the [printers? word missing] and will assist you in making the most oeconomical agreement as to paper and press work, wh sometimes is charged very exorbitantly. It seems odd that the Irish students do not graduate at their own university. You did well to pay attention to young Lettsom and should strive to cultivate his acquaintance as it may pave the way for an introduction to his father—a circumstance that may one day prove beneficial to your settling. As some time must elapse before you can be established, the sooner it is, perhaps, the better, and the sooner you will be in the way of reimbursement—an object of no small importance to your kind parent as well as to yourself. Till you are perfectly established, you'll see daily more and more reason for adhering to the strictest rules of oeconomy. The wary North Britons greatly outdo the English in this, and by this it is that they often supplant their English competitors and make their way rapidly in every part of England, nay of the globe. To assist merit struggling with difficulties wou'd at all times afford me the most exalted pleasure. But the inclination without the ability is truly painful! My losses last yr on X's Bank; on private securities, and a Chany suit now pending are more heavy than I choose to express to everyone. But independent of this, cou'd you wish me again to incur the displeasure of yr mother and brother? Before, when in compliance with yr request I lent you £10 of w[h] I could not doubt y[r] having acquainted 'em, they testified, as soon as they understood this, the utmost surprise, saying they both had and would send you the needful. Indeed I was sorry to find that what I had done hurt their minds and their laudable spirit of independence, w[h] at the same time I could not but admire. Having no doubts of y[r] friends send[g] what is necess[y] nor of your passing the tribunal with honor, I shall scarcely expect to hear f[m] you again till you appear. The portmanteau will hold y[r] clothes & a few vol[s]. Heavy books or luggage best to be shipped for Bristol. D[r] Sir, y[rs] assuredly

A. Fothergill

[1] See letter **30**, note 1.
[2] "As it seems to me".
[3] "*Pace* the learned professor".
[4] "With due deference to the learned preceptor".

N[o] 35 **36**

Bath June 5th 1794

My dear Sir

Had your former letter intimated your kind intention of addressing y[r] inaug[l] dissertation to me, I cou'd have answered it in my last, franked by Sir J. Sinclair, and forward[d] ab[t] 20th last Month w[h] I hope you have since received tho' not before your last sent out. Resolving not to bias your voluntary inclination, I have been silent on this head. Your favour of yesterday disclosing y[r] intention, I accept it with pleasure as a fresh instance of that gratitude and attention w[h] animates all your letters. Your annexing the name of my much esteemed friend D[r] Hawes gives me additional pleasure as I hope it may redound to y[r] interest, and is exactly what I should have recommended to your consideration, but for the reason above mentioned, being besides one of the properest persons (considering y[r] subject) that cou'd have been suggested. Behold this moment a letter from him wherein he writes his titles thus and desires me to communicate them to you, but I wish he had (as he perhaps has) written more fully to you

William Hawes M:D:
Sen[r] Phys[n] to the Surry and Lon[n] Dispensaries
Hon[y] Member of the R.P.S. Edin[r]: Mass H.S.
Manchester L.P.S. etc[1] — w[h] appear to me not very intelligible. Should you send him any packet you can enclose any letter etc. to me in it, as he will send me down the Philosophical Transactions some time before the end of the month. I am pleased to hear of your progress and that thus far you have passed muster with credit. My last will I hope facilitate y[r] cause till you reach the "summos in med. honores."[2] In ans[r] to your request concern[g] my titles, they are as follows. A. Fothergill — M.D., F.R.S.
Member of the Royal College of Phys[n] of London;
Honorary Member of the Medical Societies of London, Edinburgh, and Paris.
Also of the Philosophical Societies of Manchester; Philadelphia etc.[3]
Which may be abbreviated without being rendered unintelligible.

Sh'd you incline to have a motto what think you of the following?
"Phoebe, fave: novus ingreditur tua templa sacerdos"—Tibullus[4]
vel—"Multum adhuc restat operis" — Seneca[5]
vel—"Nulla re homines propius accedunt ad deos quam salutem hominibus dando"—Cicero[6]
Whatever theses connected with the subject you can procure will be interesting.

I am happy to hear your mother has got so favorably thro' a most dangerous disease and remain with best wishes for your success at this critical moment. Dr Sir, yours assuredly

A. Fothergill

[1] Woodforde's dedication read: "Necnon Viro Praestantissimo GULIELMO HAWES, M.D. Londinensi Valitudinar. Londinens. et Surrien. Med. Seniori. Societ. Reg. Phys. Edin. Soc. Honor. Societ. Human. Mancunien. et Societ. Phys. Londin. Socio. Ob urbanitatem limitissimam et amicitiam sinceram, quibus sese constanter et generose prosequi suit dignatus".

[2] "The highest honours in medicine".

[3] Woodforde's dedication read: "Viro Doctissimo et Ingeniosissimo ANTONIO FOTHERGILL, M.D. Soc. Reg. Societ. Col. Med. Reg. Londin. Soc. Societ. Medic. Londin. Edinen. et Parisien. Soc. Honor. et etiam Societ. Philosoph. Mancunien. Philadelphien., &c. Socio. Qui artem Hippocraticam, summa cum laude sua, summoque cum generis humani commodo, Bathoniae exercet; Ut indicium animi in eum, ob amicitiam benevolentiamque fere paternas, in sese, numerosissimis in exemplis, clare evidenterque demonstratas, gratissimi".

[4] "Phoebus, be favorable: a new priest enters your temples". Tibullus, *Elegies*, 2.5.1.

[5] "Much still remains to be done". Seneca, *Moral letters to Lucilius*, 64.7.

[6] "By no achievement do men come nearer to the gods than by giving health to men". Cicero, *Pro quinto lugario*, 38. Woodforde actually chose this motto (in Latin) for his thesis.

N° 38 **37**

Bath 7ber [September] 6th 1794

My dear Dr

Your affectionate letter gave me much satisfaction, and I cannot sufficiently commend your resolution of employing your leisure hours in useful study. By this, you'll be still adding to your present stock of knowledge, and having laid a good foundation will be able to carry on the superstructure with increasing pleasure. I wrote immediately to our friend Dr Hawes who probably by this time has answered your query respecting the papers. Your thesis I know he has recd, as I hope to see him ere long I shall remind him of that and other matters. From a sheet which he sent me about 10 days ago I understood his new vol. was printed off except the errata.[1] Wishing to introduce you to my esteemed friend Dr Renaudet,[2] I return his pamphlet[3] thro' yr hands with the enclosed letter which also affords you a perusal of this American tract.[4] The ensuing week I shall probably pass sometime with Dr Townsend[5] at Pewsy or perhaps in London, and have some chat with him in your behalf. Mr Dawson, as you will see from the enclosed, I have engaged warmly in your interest, and as he comes to your fair, I intend he shall be the bearer of this. So you see we are all plotting how to do you all the mischief we can. Your thesis I am circulating among medical dons, not forgetting to abuse the author as he deserves. But to be serious, on my return I shall be glad to see you whenever you can make it convenient. With best respects to yr affectionate mother and brother. I am my Dr Dr much yrs

A. Fothergill

Mr Dawson will forward this in my absence tho' he should not attend the fair which now seems uncertain. Perhaps I may be detained till about the 25th. This however is luckily the dead calm at Bath when even the turnspits stand <u>still</u>

[1] Possibly, William Hawes, *Transactions of the Royal Humane Society [from 1774 to 1784. With an appendix of miscellaneous observations on suspended animation, to . . . 1794. Edited by W. Hawes]*, [London, 1795].

[2] Peter Renaudet (1745?–?), MD (Aberdeen), practised in Bath and Bristol, Hotwells.

[3] Probably a pamphlet belonging to, not written by, Renaudet, since he seems never to have published anything.

[4] Possibly the tract by James Mease. See letter **26**, note 2.

[5] Wallis and Wallis, letter **1**, note 2, identify only one Townsend as a physician practising at this time. Richard Townsend (1740?–?), MD (Edinburgh), practised in Cork.

N° 36 **38**

Bath 28th Sep^{tr} 1794

D^{r} D^{r}

I was fav'd with y^{r} lett^{r} by Mr Bush and shall expect you here according to promise tomorrow evening, and have a bed at your service. On Tuesday about half past 3 you'll dine with me, and I shall invite Dr Moodie[1] and B. Dawson to meet you. Mr Bush bro^{t} 5 theses w^{h} you kindly sent me, but I am unwilling to deprive you of them beyond a perusal when leisure offers, after w^{h} you may have the whole or a part back with your books w^{h} were left here. Being detained with a sick friend at Highgate longer than I expected, I did not return home till Thursday last, tho' much wanted. You did right to send your thesis to D^{r} L[ettsom] and son, who, with Dr Hawes, will on my account be ready to serve you whenever occasion offers, as will Dr Renaudet who is a sincere, friendly man, but valetudinary and afraid to stir abroad—of your future plan more when we meet.

My best respects to your mother and brother and believe me, Dear Sir, yours assuredly

<u>A. Fothergill</u>

[1] Probably John Moodie (1762–1819?), MD (Aberdeen), practised at the Bath dispensary.

N° 37 **39**

Bath Octr 19th 1794

I forward this book, my D^{r} D^{r}, thro' your hands for two reasons. 1st to give you an opportunity of hasty perusal (for it must be a rapid one as Dr Renaudet himself has not yet read it) and 2^{y} that by waiting on the D^{r} with it you may improve y^{r} acquaintance with one who is so worthy our esteem. I regretted your sudden <u>escape</u> from hence before we had time to talk over affairs, and without even a sight of the Humane Society's highly finished

Medal.[1] But of these more when we meet tho' I know not when I shall be able to see you at Bristol. I hope your mother and brother are both well and have barely time to add that I am Dr Sir,

much yours
A. Fothergill

[1] Fothergill received the Humane Society's prize for an essay on suspended animation in 1794. Anthony Fothergill, *A new inquiry into the suspension of vital action, in cases of drowning and suffocation. Being an attempt . . . to elucidate the approximate cause and to appretiate* [sic] *the present remedies, and to point out the best method of restoring animation*, Bath, S. Hazard, 1795.

N° 39 **40**

Bath Octr 29th 1794

D^{r} D^{r}

Your M.S. with your obliging letter of last night came safe. What with correcting the press, composing, revising etc., added to my other engagements my hands at present are full, but if I can steal short intervals to look over your M.S. within the time, I will. And I want to make you acquainted with a worthy friend of mine and eminent practitioner who may chance some time or other to be useful to you—behold the enclosed is your introduction. My edit^{n} of Hoffmann not being the latest, viz. 1761,[1] I hastily, sometime ago, parted with it, my de Haen consists of some parts of his Ratio Medendi[2] w^{h} I never was able to anything near complete, otherwise you should have had them sent with this. But doubtless you may easily have the perusal of either at the Bristol Lib^{y} or of some of the faculty, perhaps of Dr Renaudet or Mr Baynton.[3] A scene of hurry prevents my getting thro' your Cullen M.S. and a list of anat^{y}, but if you want them only say and they shall be sent. As your mother hinted many weeks ago, her being ready to replace the sum I lent you, it will be doubly acceptable if she can do it next week, or even when you come over, as I shall want to complete a small sum against the middle of Novr due to a correspondent. Suppose you sleep here the evening before you proceed to London. On rec^{g} the Medal, being politely asked to think of a question for the next prize for 1795, I contrived to bring forward 2 which I thought might suit you to a T. So thinks friend Hawes, one would think we had been plotting. Behold one of the 2 is syncope from profuse haemorrhage. In great haste, dear D^{r}, yours

A. Fothergill

[1] Friedrich Hoffmann, *Medicinae rationalis systematicae; or, Opera omnia physico-medica denuo revisa, correcta et aucta, in sex tomos distributa, quibus continentur doctrinae solidis principiis physico-mechanicis, et anatomicis, atque etiam observationibus clinico-practicis superstructae. . . . Cum vita auctoris [by J. H. Schultze] et ejus praefatione de differente medicinae et medicorum statu*, 6 vols. in 3, Geneva, de Tournes, 1761.

[2] Anton de Haën (1704–1776), *Ratio medendi nosocomio practico, quod . . . condidit Maria Theresia . . . Imperatrix*, 5 vols., Vienna, J. T. von Trattner; H. Krüchten, 1760–67.

[3] Thomas Baynton (1761–1820), surgeon at Bristol, developed a method for treating ulcers of the legs. See letter **55**.

N° 41 **41**

[Bath December 1794]

D^r^ D^r^

Pursuant to y^r^ request no time has been lost in adding my testimony to y^r^ credentials. Preserve a fair copy of my letter w^h^ I trust may avail you on more occasions than the present, and perhaps carry more weight than a whole cargo of random recommendations from persons less competent to judge. As M^r^ D[awson] joins me heartily in y^r^ interest and is intimate with Mrs Beck's uncle, he promised me to wait on him this day to entreat him to write to his niece in your favour. Y^r^ lett^r^ will explain tho' occasion the shortness of time. Whether you succeed or not in your present application, the ardor of y^r^ friends will not fail to cause others to embark in y^r^ interest, and ensure y^r^ establishment. My respects to Dr Renaudet and Mr Baynton, and you'll do well to consult 'em on this occasion. You'll wait on the Governors in person, and, if from home, leave a respectful card intreating the favor of their vote and interest.[1]

Health and success

adieu A. Fothergill

Bath Dec^r^: ult: 94

[1] Woodforde was obviously a candidate for an appointment at a voluntary hospital, possibly the Bristol Royal Infirmary.

N° 40 **42**

Bath Jany 27th 1795

D^r^ D^r^

Herewith I hope you'll receive safe Hippocrates and Aretaeus[1] two of the most venerable of the ancients, and w^h^ it is strange the Bristol Lib^y^ sh^d^ be without, tho' most provincial Lib^ys^ are miserably defective in med^l^ authors. These, with the voluminous authors you mention, if perused with care, as they must be if read to advantage, will engross all y^r^ leisure hours for this very considerable time to come. However I send them without delay to be in readiness. The printer and I meet with so many interruptions that my press work goes on but slowly, tho' we are got to the 80th page, and it will not be my fault if the rest be not expedited. Being ever too nice in correction and attempts towards improvement, I find the revision[2] not a work of recreation–but of re-creation. The case you describe seems to be a real suppuration of the liver, and if it breaks externally by emoll^t cataplasms etc. and you can keep air from penetrating the abdomen, all may still do well, tho' a very critical situation of w^h the man's relatives should be privately admonished. It will be right to take notes as you pass thro' the above important authors. Remember me kindly to Dr Renaudet, Mr Baynton etc

D^r D^r, yours in great haste
A. Fothergill

P.S. When you next come to Bath bring with you the M.S. of College exercises I sent you to Edin^r[3]

[1] Presumably one of the many editions of Aretaeus of Cappadocia (AD *c.*150–200, *De causis et signis acutorum et diuturnorum morborum.*

[2] There does not seem to have been any new editions of any of Fothergill's works in 1795, so what is being discussed here is unclear. He was probably referring to the manuscript of of his *Inquiry*, see letter **39**, note 1.

[3] See letters **27, 32** and **46**.

N° 42 **43**

Bath April 10th 1795

D^r D^r

Daily journeys to country patients in addition to my other numerous avocations have put it out of my power to ans^r y^r last oblig^g fav^r with the loan of Fordyce's book[1] till now. I am happy, however, to hear y^r late visit to Bath afforded not only consolation to y^r mind, then under great agitation, but a truce to y^r bodily complaints, besides sparing you the expense and inconvenience of being long absent from home. If the slight glut w^h still recurs at intervals be divested of all virulence and contagion (as I trust it is) the vessels, if not too much urged and irritated by astrigent stimulants, will in due time recover their tone. Instead of harassing the mucous membrane with injections of this kind, suppose you leave the matter to the powers of the system; gently aiding these by the cold bath treatment[?] or a cold water fall from the height of 4 or 5 feet, on the genitals every morn^g—taking 4 or 6 pills of G: Oliban:[2] with [antimony symbol] of P. Rh[?]i every night.[3] As soon as a leisure hour will permit I will run over Dr Fordyce on Simple Fevers[4] and return it safe. The printer thro' absurd forgetfulness instead of working off some extra copies of my Inq^y as ordered, expressly in the presence of the compositor and pressmen, only printed just the Society's number.[5] Hence I am left with 2 imperfect copies for myself, one of w^h I request y^r acceptance of herewith, which being much disguised with corrections is only fit for your private perusal, tho' sufficiently legible. Wishing you success in your new situation, I remain D^r D^r in haste much yours

A. Fothergill

[1] Possibly one of many editions of George Fordyce (1736–1802), *Elements of the practice of physic. Part the I. Containing, the natural history of the human body. Part the II. Containing, the history and methods of*

treating fevers, and internal inflammations, London, J. Johnson, 1771. Sixth edition, 1791.

2 Olibanum is sometimes described as a gum and sometimes as a resin. It is also known as frankincense.

3 The symbol is that of antimony and the prescription makes no sense. It probably should read, take "oliban with antimony [possibly meaning tartar emeticus] and P. Rh[?]i". The latter could be Rhaei, an unusual spelling for rhubarb root, or Rhoei which could refer to wild poppy. The former is most likely.

4 George Fordyce, *A dissertation on simple fever, or on fever consisting of one paroxysm only*, London, J.Johnson, 1794.

5 See letter **39**, note 1.

N° 43 **44**

Bath June 3rd 179[5] [figure illegible]

Dear Sir,

I am happy to find that your health and spirits are so well restored and that you enjoy once more the greatest of sublunary blessings, the

"Mens sana in corpore sano."[1]

Mrs Woodforde's request alas! happens at a most unfortunate time, for on Friday last I parted with what ready cash I had to spare, in a remittance to Londn to the amount of 40£. Indeed since my late villain of a servant by means of a false key stole several Gs out of my escritoire, I have made a point of keeping by me only small sums for current expenses. Add to this Mr Chaplin, who had promised to pay in a sum on mortgage on Monday last 1st June, writes that his correspondt has disappointed him, so behold the payment is put off sine die!!!—Dreadful times! no punctuality of payment—increasing burthens and decreasing ability to support them, and yet in spite of all this, people of all ranks live beyond their incomes, and by lighting the candle at both ends quickly exhaust every resource, and plunge themselves into bankruptcy! The small sum wanted however for present exigency will no doubt soon be raised by your brother among some of the monied Bristolians. By the by, if any of his clients will advance me 600£ on an undoubted security of a mortgage on a leasehold estate near Bath on 3 good lives, interest at 5 per cent which is punctually paid half yearly, I shall then be able to supply Mrs Woodforde with the sum you mention. Time and assiduity as I formerly admonished you must be required to gain you a firm establishment especially among so many hungry antagonists. Your prospect however, for the time is superior to most of the juvenile physicians. Your tract of Fordyce's I passed thro' the hands of good Renaudet who has or will convey it to you safely, and your other books I shall now hasten thro' and return in due time. Best respects to your dear mother and brother and believe me, Dear Sir,

yrs assuredly
A. Fothergill

P:S: I think you have my late tract on the poison of lead and copper etc.[2] or I would send you a copy. No copies alas! on Vital Action[3] but what I must buy, as lately one for Phill Socy of Philadelphia wh I forwarded by the hands of Dr Renaudet, to whom my best respects and who will, I hope, not forget his long promised visit to Bath accompanied with fresh dispatches from his worthy nephew Judge Turner, of wh his late short letter gave intimation and for wh I wait with the utmost impatience. Vale! P.S. The messenger who brot yrs neglecting to wait or call in half an hour for the ans[r] obliges me to forward this by the coach, after waiting a day his promised return.

[1] "A healthy mind in a healthy body". Juvenal, *Satires*, 10.356.
[2] See letter **6**, note 6. Fothergill actually used the symbols derived from alchemy to indicate the metals.
[3] See letter **39**, note 1.

N° 44 **45**

Bath June 18th 1795

Dear Sir

After mature consideration of your patient's history, it is still by no measure clear either from the remote cause assigned or from the symptoms, whether the irritating cause is seated in the encephalon, or the stomach or the duodenum. As the menses are reg[r] we cannot fairly attribute the origin of the disease to the effects of damp linen. Worms in the alimentary canal have more than once caused similar affections. With this view, and also to get rid of the mercur[l] sympt[s], I shou'd be inclined to try the following plan about 3 weeks; if it fails, the succeeding ones may deserve attention. Charge her to observe all her stools—to leave off tea and never make a full meal. With best wishes for your success in this obscure case, and all others committed to your care, I remain

D[r] D[r] in haste much y[rs]
A: Fothergill

P:S: My respects to D[r] Renaudet, M[r] Baynton etc. I hope M[rs] W[oodforde] got the [money? illegible] without difficulty.

N° 46 **46**

Bath Sept[r] 19th 1794 [1795][1]

My D[r] Sir,

Your kind mother has my best thanks for a couple fine chickens w[h] arrived here this morning in my absence with M[c]bride's Practice,[2] and am sorry the messenger left no word where he was to be found, or whether inclined to bring an ans[r]. The only M.S. returned with former parcel was a Latin case, and I have turned over Hippocrates and Aretaeus from beginning to end, but the Ordo Examin:[3] so much wanted is not to be found, tho' it is to be hoped your Edin[r] correspond[t] if it has been lent out will yet recover it. In the progress of my inquiry on y[r] account I have just heard that a vacancy of a physic[n] to Northamp[n] hospital has been lately announced in the Lond[n] papers, but doubtless numerous medical candidates all around will crowd forwards, add to this D[r] Curry of Kettering[4] well known at Northhampton from former residence, will probably supersede all others, having been employed some time ago by the directors of the new Humane Society established at Northampton to draw up a short statement of the method to be pursued, w[h] he performed much to their satisfaction. To cope with Kerr[5] who rules with unrivaled sway it wou'd require that an antagonist should appear flush of money with a couple of good saddle horses, a livery serv[t] and other things in style to please this proud, showy, dressy people, who weigh medical mind by external appearances—a plan where an Akenside,[6] a Stonhouse,[7] a Watts,[8] a Kerr etc. have been accustomed to set every engine to work, and to push on business by machinery. This would not suit you. The expedition forming for the West Ind[s] will demand a number of med[l] and chirurg[l] attendants but I know of no key to these military commanders who fix the appointments, otherwise a good introduction to practice might thus be obtained. Your brother in Lond[n] might by diligent application and inquiry at the respective offices in Lond[n] obtain the necess[y] intelligence and you might send a letter to the board setting forth the course of your studies and your readiness to embark in the service provided you should feel an inclination to undertake a western voyage. Without some speedy exertion of this sort, you may, it is fear'd, remain a considerable time longer unknown, unemployed. To obviate this and to forward your wishes is the ardent desire of

Dear Sir,
Yours very sincerely
A. Fothergill

P.S. Beddoes edit[n] of Brown[9] has not found its way into the Bath libraries as yet.

[1] The reference to Beddoes's edition of John Brown, see this letter note 9, along with other evidence, dates this as 1795.

[2] David Macbride (1726–1778), *A methodical introduction to the theory and practice of physic*, London, W. Strahan, 1772.

[3] Fothergill seems to be referring here to the catechism he sent to Woodforde in Edinburgh. See letters **27**, **32** and **42**.

[4] Presumably James Curry (1755–1819), MD (Edinburgh 1784), FSA, became physician to the County hospital (Northampton), later removed to London, Licentiate of the College of Physicians (1802), and eventually physician to Guy's Hospital.

[5] Presumably William Kerr (1738–1824), MD (Oxford), Army surgeon and surgeon to the Infirmary at the County Hospital (Northampton), later he practised as a physician in Northampton.

[6] Presumably Mark Akenside (1721–1770), poet and physician, doctor of physic (Leyden 1744), FRS, FCP.

[7] Sir James Stonhouse. See letter **8**, note 3.

[8] Presumably William Watts (1725–1786), MD (Aberdeen), practised in Northampton.

[9] John Brown (1735–1788), *The elements of medicine. Translated from the Latin, with comments and illustrations, by the author. A new ed. . . . with a biographical preface by Thomas Beddoes*, 2 vols., London, J. Johnson, 1795.

N[o] 45 **47**

Bath Nov: 25th 1795

Dear Sir

My friend Kingston kindly called just now with the enclosed letter from his correspond[t]

in London whom he wrote purposing on y^r account. I therefore forward it without delay for y^r information. The place he presumes is still vacant as no intelligence has arrived of its being filled. From this account together with information you collect f^m y^r Bristol correspond^ce, you'll learn whether a successor has gone over, and to form a judgement of its eligibility. You will of course consult y^r friends and from the general result form your determination. All I know of the matter is now before you. Sh^d you wish to consult Dr Kingston again, he is removed f^m N° 16 to No 20 Milsom street. Madeira belongs to the crown of Portugal, and except the English factory and English sojourners, the inhabitants are Portuguese, hence the restriction about dispensing med^s. Tho' the Portuguese have physic^s of their own, yet they generally give preferences to an English practitioner and that for very wise reasons. They are better instructed. I remain, Dr Sir, in haste much yours

A. Fothergill

P.S. How far the present locum tenens is likely to prove an antagonist you'll judge f^m the letter.

[N° 88a] **48**

Copy of a letter received from Mr Jas Russell Surgeon, Edin^r.[1]

16th of December 1795

Dr Sir,

I am favored with y^r letter of 10th ins in which you do me the honor to ask my advice for a young relation who unhappily has been deprived of the sight of both eyes by an attack of cataract. By the account given of the case there seems to be nothing remarkable in the appearance of the eyes, nor any thing in the state of the symptoms unfavorable to an operation so that the time of operating is the only point to be determined. Now it is plain that it never can be adviseable to operate till the eye be so large and the patient so steady as to allow all the steps of the operation to be performed with tolerable certainty of success and these circumstances cannot be expected to take place sooner than 8 or 10 years of age; tho' more probably not till 12 or 14. About 12 therefore I consider as the medium line of life at w^h the operation of couching is performed, there is a chance that the state of the eye and of the patient's steadiness may admit of operating a year or two sooner. But if extraction is to be performed, 12 will be in all likelihood the earliest age at w^h the operation will be adviseable, I sh^d not however esteem it prudent to determine a particular case by a general rule; without taking into consideration all the specialities in the patient's situation. Upon this account I sh^d recommend the occasional examination of his eyes when the period of life approaches at w^h it may be prudent to perform the operation in order that the surgeon may avail himself of the first favourable opportunity to attempt to restore him to sight. As to the operation w^h I prefer, I have in general given the preference to depression, though I do not think the preference very marked and sh^d think that if y^r own inclination leads you to prefer extraction you ought undoubtedly to recommend it to y^r relation. There is one advantage attends depression in this case: it can probably be admitted some years sooner, w[h] is so much time gained in the acquisition of knowledge. Whatever you determine on I shall be glad to learn the result of the operation. I sincerely hope it will be favourable and I do assure you it will give me the greatest pleasure to think that my advice can be of use to you either on this or any other occasion. I remain D[r] Sir y[r] most obd[t] and very humble servant.

James Russell

P.S. My friend's letter is very pertinent and satisfactory but I cou'd wish he had been more definite in mentioning when the eye became large enough for performing an operation. If the full growth of the eye is requisite this cannot take place before the age 18 or 20. The chief impediments in my opinion to the early performing [of] the operation are the unsteadiness of the patient and of course the inability of the surgeon to perform properly the several steps of the operation. Were proper instruments contrived for fixing the eye at pleasure—why may not the operation be performed at a very early age? I sh[d] suppose the eye not more susceptible at 2 or 3 years of age than at 12 or 14. And all agree in affirming that it is the consequent inflammation w[h] usually frustrates the cure. But probably the force that wou'd be requisite to fix the eye without any cooperation of the patient wou'd excite inflammation. This to me is the only reason why we may not immediately attempt to restore vision. Since writing the above it occurs to me that puberty takes place in each sex about the age of 10 or 14 years, but the body has not acquired its full and perfect growth at this time. Dr Gregory fixes this to about the 18th or 20th year.

"Justam et plenam staturam juvenis forsan adipiscitur decimo octavo vel vigesimo ætatis anno."[2] Since Mr Russell's letter I have been honored with the opinion of two other eminent practitioners in surgery: Mr Fyfe[3] and Mr Latta.[4] Mr Fyfe thinks extraction better than couching. Mr Latta prefers the latter and both agree in considering it improper to operate before the eyes are of such growth, and the patient so sensible and steady as to allow all the steps of the operation to be properly performed.

[1] James Russell (1754–1836) was an Edinburgh surgeon, author and first professor of clinical surgery at the university, 1803. This letter is unnumbered. It appears in the letterbook after letter N° 88 (**87** in this sequence), the last from Philadelphia and before the final two letters from London, N° 89 and N° 90 (**90** and **91** in this sequence). We have numbered it 88a to locate it in the letterbook but placed it chronologically as **48** in this sequence. It seems that the original from Russell was sent to Fothergill who then sent it to Woodforde with a P.S.

[2] "A young man reaches his proper full stature perhaps in his eighteenth or twentieth year". Not attributable.

[3] Presumably Andrew Fyfe (1754–1824), anatomist, dissector to Alexander Monro, *secundus*, professor of anatomy in the university of Edinburgh. See letter **20**, note 1.

[4] Presumably James Latta (1765?–1804), FRCSE, surgeon-apothecary in Edinburgh, and author of *A practical system of surgery*, 3 vols., Edinburgh, G. Mudie, A. Guthrie & J. Fairbairn, 1795.

N° 48 **49**

Bath Apr 26 (Tues Even) [1796][1]

Watchful, my dear Sir, for y^{r} interest, I seize the earliest opportunity of acquainting you that there is a vacancy of physic^{n} to the Salisbury Infirmary just declared in consequence of Dr Dobson's resignation and quitting the profession and that the elect^{n} will come on about a fortnight hence. Consequently if you think it wou'd ans^{r} y^{r} purpose, no time ought to be lost. Dr Grove[2] is the other sen^{r} resident physic^{n} but relinquishing the Infirmary long ago. Dr Barlow is gone to the West Ind^{s} and his return doubtful, so that the place, at present, seems to present a promising opening for a phys^{n} especially if he succeeds at the Infirmary. Such is the opinion of Dr Dobson whom I met yest^{y} on the case of a young lady about 12 miles from Salisbury and who promised to pay attention to any candidate whom I sh^{d} recommend. Dr Harvey, late of Holt now of Wincanton, has connections with the Everetts and the leading persons in the neighbourhood, and has this day (on meeting him casually in Bath) promised, if you settle and will call on him, he will at my request, to give you recommend^{y} letters to the Everetts etc. I have also endeav^{d} to engage Mr Seagram, surg^{n}, in y^{r} interest. From the above you will learn my opinion, but as I have always said, in a matter of such moment, I cannot, dare not advise. From comparing circumstances on a view of the place and consulting your friends you may perhaps be able to form a judgement. Subscribers are requested to withhold all promise of their votes till the day of election—a prudent measure and probab^{y} suggested by the Earl of Radnor. Thus all may start fair. No honor lost by application—tho' the candidate fails of success. Your Brown's Elements and Hamilton's Morgagni[3] arrived before Mr Townsend's departure and safe here Dear Sir, With best respects to your mother}
sorry I was out when you called} yours assuredly
being a week in London} A. Fothergill

P.S. If you resolve to reconnoitre the town you may call on Dr Dobson with freedom (to whom I have opened the matter) and learn every particular. One saddle horse will at least be necessary if you settle at Salisbury, a very genteel town and opulent neighbourhood. But strict oeconomy these times must be the maxim throughout England. Dr Dobson has heard of no candidate yet, except a Dr Baker,[4] and thinks this need be no discouragement to others as he hints that he makes 600 per annum in his present and therefore seems indifferent. I have now given you all I know on the subject and have only to add my best wishes. I shall meet Dr Dobson again at Boyton[5] to see Miss Lambert on Thursday. Vale!

[1] The following letter (**50**) refers to the Salisbury vacancy, dating this one as 1796.

[2] Charles Grove (1747–1806), MD (St. John's College, Cambridge), physician to Salisbury Hospital.

[3] James Hamilton (1767–1839), *Observations on the seats and causes of disease; illustrated by the dissections of the late professor Morgagni of Padua*, vol.1, Edinburgh, 1795. No more published.

[4] Possibly Thomas Baker (1755–?), MD (Oxford?), practised in Bath, Norwich, and Leighton Buzzard, Bedfordshire.

[5] Boyton, a parish near Trowbridge, Wiltshire.

N° 47 **50**

Bath May 25th 1796

Dear Sir

During my absence from home arrived your obliging present of 4 chickens, one of which was the same night secretly conveyed from my garden, supposed to be effected by some rapacious cat. As the basket was ordered to wait here I shall, when Mr Townsend comes over, which I expect will be some time before the end of June, return it with y^{r} books by the carrier. By whom the vacancy at Salisbury is filled I have not heard, but think on the whole you determined wisely as it cou'd not (admitting you had carried it in preference to the other candidates of which there might have been much doubt) have been occupied without considerable expense at the offset. To carry an election for a hosp^{l} or even dispens^{y} in London, often costs the candidate from 500 to 1000$^{£}$ sterling. Some of these have a small salary annexed, others not, and in the country, except Haslar and Plymouth, I know not of one that has any salary—candidates always in plenty who offer their service <u>gratis</u>. Besides the multiplicity of other charities continually starting up, tends to divest the current of subscriptions, by w^{h} most of the hosp^{ls} are reduced to a low ebb, and find difficulty to keep their doors open to the wonted number of petitioning invalids. The numerous dispensaries have contributed not a little to the above defalcations, and have at the same time materially injured medical and chirurg^{l} practitioners and subtracted considerably from their annual resources. As soon as you are doing well at Castle Cary and have a large scope of country free from competitors, and live almost without expense, I cannot see why you may not in time extend y^{r} present sphere and render it productive of a very handsome income, perhaps superior to that of a large town with 3 or 4 senior antagonists. If you set apart 2 hours every day in prescribing for paupers they will not fail to spread your fame, and bring in opulent farmers and by degrees the neighbour^{g} gentry. But to do this [you] must sit down resolutely bent to continue, for if the slightest hint escapes you of a design to relinquish, it will at once destroy the interest you have made and damp all future hopes of establish^{t} among them. Dr Pulteney at Blandford[1] and other eminent men have done exceedingly well in small, insignificant, country towns. It is not the mere town that is an object but a populous neighbourhood and expanse of country unoccupied. An independency in physic is not to be obtained in these times without patient perseverance and indefatigable diligence for a course of years. The heavy expense of a great country [practice] is a grievous drawback and keeps many young practitioners of merit in a state of penury thro' life. If you obtain the interest of the apoth^{s} of the neighbour^{g} towns it will be a material step gained. Next to these you must gain over the clergy, school masters, midwives etc. etc. Dr Hawes J^{ur} displays much ingenuity and acumen in his Morgagni and I shall be glad to see the sequel. At present you may hire a horse cheaper than keep one w^{h} requires a serv^{t} to take care of him. In all difficult cases propose a senior physician in consult^{n} who, if he has y^{r} interest at heart as I have, he may rivet y^{r} interest. With best respects to y^{r} kind mother, with thanks for her present. I remain, D^{r} D^{r}

y^{r} assured friend
<u>A. Fothergill</u>

Anthony Fothergill

[1] Richard Pulteney (1730–1801), MD (Edinburgh 1764), FRSE, FLS, Extra-Licentiate of the RCP (1765), apothecary and physician, practised in Blandford, Dorset.

N° 51 **51**

Bath Octr 29th 1796

Dr Sir,

Herewith I hope you'll receive safe Brown's Elemt^{s}, 4 vols., Hamilton's Morgagni; 1 vol. with your M.S. cases—for the perusal of w^{h} accept my thanks. Had I not waited for Mr Townsend and your promised journey to Bath the parcel wou'd have been dispatched much sooner. Respecting Wry's case w^{h} you have well explained I know not whose care he is under in the Bath Hosp^{l} but I fear the prostate gland and cervix vesicæ[1] are indurated. Warm bathing, electr^{y} and blister to the lumbar region with Aq: Nephrit: alcal:[2] with milk internally might, I should hope, administer relief. In Abraham's case—the sensorial power is intercepted in some branches of the dorsal nerves and from this torpor–irreg^{r} motions are excited in other organs. Here, pumping of B:T: on the loins[3]—electr^{y} and blister[ing] are clearly indicated.

Internally T: Gucaci: vols 3 drachms T: Opii g^{r} xx—bis die aa [?]: e Lignis.[4]

The case of haematuria is extremely well explained and judiciously treated. The contusion of the kidney injured the secretion and gave a tendency to gravellish concretions. Next to rigid abstinence—on which I should place most stress—wou'd be alvine laxatives to produce piles or determin^{ns} to the hæmor^{l} vessels to disburthen the renal.

I was lately consulted together with Dr Crane[5] on the subdean's case at Wells; a periodical idiopathic haematuria—past the meridian of life and bon vivant—plethoric and sedentary. Has had 4 attacks in about 10 years—by similar plan has always found relief.

I am glad to hear y^{r} practice increases and agree with you in full conviction that a country station affords all the superior advantages respecting health, study etc., you mention. Respecting fees—moderation is the safest and most political side to lean to. I lately borrowed Zoonomia[6] at the Lib^{y} and run it hastily over. It exhibits an intermediate system between Cullen and Brown with improvement on the former and without the extravagancies of the latter. Much ingenuity however with no small portion of eccentricity. But it sh^{d} be read 2 or 3 times before a critical opinion can be formed, and half a century must elapse before the system can be expected to be adopted, and many revisions before it can be perfected. I perused Mr Hamilton's Morgagni with much pleasure, but with the orig^{l} or Alexander translation[7] being in most student's hands, I wish he had given an orig^{l} work on dissections with histories of cases prefixed without confining himself wholly to Morgagni. Morgagni's cases of pyrexia are by no means so clearly marked as might be wished. To reduce his rude matter into order according to modern pathology is a most arduous undertaking. Were accurate histories and dissections recorded at all our hospitals, a most important work might in time be formed from the materials. At present they are too scarce and too <u>isolated</u>. Mr Hamilton, so far as he has gone, has executed his plan greatly beyond what I cou'd have expected and in his notes and observations has displayed no small share of critical acumen. I wish him all possible success—But alas! while the public mind is absorbed in politics and stunned by the din of arms scarcely any medical work how important so ever and tho' written with a sunbeam would be sufficient to command attention—much less remunerate the author. With best respects to M[rs] Woodforde I remain,

Dear Sir, much yours,

A. Fothergill

P.S. When you come this way or forward any packet, pray don't forget to send Lettsom on Tea[8] and the other little tracts, some of which a friend or 2 wants to look over.

[1] The neck of the bladder.

[2] Aqua Nephritica had nutmeg as its principal ingredient. Alcal. possibly refers to an alkali, i.e. potash or soda.

[3] We have been unable to clarify this.

[4] Fothergill was prescribing (in the signs for Apothecary measures) 3 drachms of Tinctura Guaiacina volatilis and 20 grains of Tincture of opium—aa—of each—to be taken—*bis die*—twice a day. e Lignis could be a reference to Nephriticum Lignum, a South American wood used as a diuretic. e Lignis is not a recognized usage however.

[5] John Crane (1760–?), physician at Dorchester.

[6] Erasmus Darwin (1731–1802), *Zoonomia; or, the laws of organic life*, 2 vols., London, J. Johnson, 1794–96.

[7] Morgagni, see letter **23**, note 7. See also letter **49**, note 3.

[8] John Coakley Lettsom, *The natural history of the tea-tree, with observations on the medical qualities of tea, and effects of tea-drinking*, London, E. & C. Dilly, 1772.

N° 49 **52**

Bath Nov 5th 1796

Accept my thanks, D[r] Sir, for your obliging present just now arrived. I am pleased to hear y[r] dear mother got home safe and has had no return of a 2nd attack which however we have still some reason to dread, espec[y] if she suffers anxiety to prey on her mind, but which she must by all possible means strive to avoid. Shou'd it unfortunately recur, shou'd recommend cupping with scarificat[n] in the nape of the neck followed by a blister immediately on the part. The cathartic to be repeated as circumstances may point out and a nasal discharge encouraged by an occasional sternutatory.[1]

The head elevated in bed by an additional pillow. Nutritive diet in moderation but never a full meal. Drink may consist of good table beer, or toast and water with a little Lisbon or old raisin wine.

You'll easily comprehend the reason of these admonitions, and from the nature of the disease, see clearly their importance. I need not be more particular as your own good sense and penetration will readily suggest the principal indications, and your filial regard and affection will prompt you to pursue them with attention. With best wishes for y[r] dear parent's perfect recovery. I remain, Dear D[r], y[rs] very sincerely.

A. Fothergill

[1] A medicine used to produce sneezing.

N° 50 **53**

[December 26] [1796?]

Dr Sir,

By accident, I this moment saw your advertisement in the Bristol paper—send me by coach or post immediately the list of subscribers that I may write to each I have any knowledge of, in your favour

Decr 26 Yours sincerely

Bath Walcot Parade N° 17 B. Dawson

P.S. To the above kind proposal, I must heartily [word missing] and you may rely on what interest we can muster. Be first well-assured of Dr W. resignation, for should the report be premature or sh^{d} he alter his mind you'll all be dished for geese, and y^{r} friends scouted for ganders. At all events, as the contest may be strong, and continue many weeks, launch not out into unnecessary expense, where the event must be uncertain and where perhaps, 2 of y^{r} opponents may unite their forces, and substitute cabal in place of merit. The Board sh'd request Governors not to promise their votes to the 1st comer but to wait till the merit of the respective candidates is well weighed, and their credentials duly examined. But the family of the wrong-heads is everywhere numerous and generally carry matter their own way, right or wrong, but more freq^{y} ye latter, being unqualified to judge. With best wishes for y^{r} success, D^{r} D^{r}, much yours

A. Fothergill

N° 62 **54**

Bath Jan: 25th /97

Dr Sir,

In daily expectation of some favorable opportunity of conveyance, I have waited till now that Mr Jean offers to deliver you this letter. In autumnal diseases and particularly in gouty habits attended with atonia, it will, I presume, be generally found that the temporary relief obtained by the lancet is on the whole dearly purchased. The dysenteric case you describe is I fear f^{m} long continuance become habitual, and the determination to the intestinal glands not easy to be removed. In some of these inveterate cases a considerable tract of the rectum and larger intestines have, on dissection, been found in a schirrous, sometimes in an ulcerated state, with considerable thickening of the intestinal coats and coarctation in certain parts of the canal. If this sh^{d} on examination with the finger be found to be the case, the disease will terminate in an incurable marasmus. If not, there may still be hopes especially if the patient cou'd go to a warm climate for 5 or 6 months, as Lisbon, Naples etc. At all events he sh^{d} wear flannel next the skin, and keep up a constant and if possible equable perspiration by mild anodyne perspiratives. The follow^{g} demulcent for common drink often proves salutary. Take of mutton suet fresh—One Apothecary ounce

—Milk—One pound or 12 Apothecary ounces
—Flour—One half Apothecary ounce
—Cinnamon—One half drachm[1]

Simmer the whole over a gentle fire about 5 minutes stirring it constantly. Leeches to the hæmorrhoids might afford temporary relief if there be throbbing and distention. The camp dysentery proceeding from marsh miasmata or putrid animal effluvia is doubtless contagious, but the present case seems not to have arisen under any suspicious circumstances of this sort, and it is supposed his domestics remain free from the disease. The malignant fever in the West Indies has, I hear, carried off since the commencement of the late ill-fated exped^{n} more than 16 med^{l} practitioners, above 200 officers and privates almost innumerable. I am pleased to reflect on y^{r} inclination of hazarding such a dangerous voyage was happily defeated, espec^{y} as I hear of y^{r} increasing success in a fine healthy rural situation free f^{m} the horrid din of arms. I am happy to hear y^{r} dear mother continues to recover, and remain with best wishes Dr Sir, much y^{rs}

P. s. No news f^{m} Mr Townsend. A. Fothergill

Dr Hawes writes that Mr Kempton, surgeon, carried his elect^{n} for London Hosp^{l} against 9 others, attended the committee and the day follow^{g} died apoplectic, aged 21.

[1] Fothergill gave the amounts in the signs for Apothecary measures.

N° 54 **55**

Bath Aug: 27th 97

Dear Sir

Your letter of yesterday did not arrive till near midnight, consequently cou'd not be ans^{d} by the Shepton carrier who sets out about noon. Being marked carriage paid, my housekeeper refused paying 9^{d}, w^{h} Pickwick's porter charges, assuring her the carriage was not paid. This you will of course explain that she knows how to act, to pay what is right, or prevent imposition. Besides the latter part of the letter implies its being sent by a messenger, not by any of the coaches. On such occasions as these never trust to anything short of an express messenger. The enclosed to Marshall I delivered this morn^{g} who was absent from home. To the many inquiries concern^{g} Mrs Purlewent w^{h} have been made since I saw her (now near 7 weeks!) I must confess I was much at a loss how to answer, and not a little surprised at your silence! From y^{r} accurate and circumstantial acc^{t} it appears that the remedies proposed, and particularly the digitalis, seemed to hold the disease at bay by subduing the hydropic symptoms, and insuring a copious flow of urine. When she grew tired of this, the disease, with its concomitant affections of the brain, gained ground, accompanied with increasing debility. That various other med^{s} have been since successively tried without the desired effect, for the increasing danger seems now to threaten a fatal termination. In a case of such infinite consequence to the patient—to her afflicted husband, and to the family! —a case w^{h} has its seat in the brain! and is in every point of view so extremely urgent!

and w[h] demands in its treatment the utmost skill and discernment, and at the same time the most prudent and vigorous measures, you must be convinced that it is impossible for me, with either justice to our patient or satisfaction to myself, to propose any new plan without being on the spot and examining the pulse, the countenance and every leading and present circumstance w[h] a quarter of an hour's observation at the bedside can alone supply, and w[h] far exceeds the most elaborate description. Please to inform M[r] Purlewent of this truth and if he inclines that we sh[d] meet and make one more vigorous effort in her favor, you'll give me timely notice, and assure him of my best, my ardent wishes to administer every possible relief in this most distressing case. In the interim I am D[r] D[r] much y[rs]

A. Fothergill

P.S. M[r] Baynton waits my remarks on his tract w[h] I lent you on ulcerated legs and delays the press for 2nd edit[n].[1] He wrote last week while I was in London. N.B. My regards to y[r] d[r] mother.

[1] Thomas Baynton, *Descriptive account of a new method of treating old ulcers of the legs*, Bristol, N. Biggs, 1797; second edition, Bristol, Emery & Adams, 1799. The P.S. seems to imply that the year was 1799, when Baynton's second edition appeared. Fothergill's regards to Woodforde's mother negate this possibility. She was dead in August 1799. The evidence of Mrs. Purlewent's case (see letter **56**) suggests 1797 as the most likely. Perhaps Baynton's *Account* had appeared very early in 1797 and he was hoping for a second edition later that year or early the next.

N° 55 **56**

Bath 8[ber] [October] 16th 1792 [1797]

Dear Sir,

I lament that your patient's case continues to baffle all your efforts. You have, it seems, tried the full force of diuretics, sudorifics and even mercury itself, whence it appears clear to me that the disease ought no longer to be treated vi et armis,[1] but that the constitution ought to be restored and the digestive organs improved by some mild restoratives, otherwise it is to be feared she will soon undergo a total prostration of strength, and get into a lingering state of hopeless debility worse than even death itself. Not long ago an epileptic girl at a neighbouring boarding school, of a feeble constitution and still weaker digestive powers attended with severe headache and giddiness. She had tried, before I saw her, sundry Herculean remedies which rather exasperated the disease. I advised a course of Bath waters, here on the spot, with mild restoratives, on w[h] she soon recovered and that without any subsequent relapse. A beautiful young lady of 15 in Portland Place labouring under similar symptoms is now going on under similar treatment with very promising signs of success. Please to communicate this to M[r] Purlewent with my best respects and acquaint him that had I an opportunity of seeing his wife (whose case I greatly pity), I should by no means despair of convincing her of the absolute necessity of beginning some plan of this kind and submitting to strict regimen, without w[h] the best plan may be defeated. To prevent loss of time and to clear the system of the remains of mercury, w^h may be done in about 3 days, I would advise the following; instead of giving way to despondency let me persuade her to cherish hope and resolve for her own sake and that of her family, to let nothing on her part be wanting that may administer to her relief or contribute to the satisfaction of her relations. With best wishes for her recovery. I am, Dr Sir, much yours.

A. Fothergill

P.S. The tracts on pneum^l medicine publ^d by Beddoes, Watt etc.,[2] are, amount^g to ab^t 14 or 15^s/- Many of the cases are now doubted. 3 numbers were lent to me to read, but I shall not purchase the rest. The Boston Amer^n Mem^s, a Micell^s work with some good papers.[3] 1st vol. I have had from Bath Agricultural Soc^y but not the rest, but of these matters more when we meet. N.B. My respects to Mrs Woodforde.

[1] "By force of arms".
[2] Thomas Beddoes (1760–1808) and James Watt (1736–1819), *Considerations on the medicinal use of factitious airs and on the manner of obtaining them*, 5 pts. in 1 vol., Bristol, Bulgin & Rosser, [1794?]–1796.
[3] *Memoirs of the American Academy of Arts and Sciences*, vols. 1–2, Boston, 1785–93.

N° 52 **57**

Bath Feb 17th 1798

Before me, Dear Sir, is your favour received a few days ago, from w^h I am much concerned to hear your dear mother has suffered another attack. However as you are in possession of the means which formerly not only afforded relief, but also procured a longer interval than cou'd well be expected, you'll be at no loss how to modify the same to present circumstances and the exigencies of the case. Should these fail I see no objection to a trial of electricity, but must observe that notwithstanding it seems so perfectly apposite to the nature of the disease and at first view holds forth the most promising hopes of relief, yet in no disease to w^h it seems adapted has it so little answered my expectation as in palsies. This among other instances ought to inspire diffidence in medical theories even when they assume the most flattering aspect. "Non fingendum aut excogitandum (says the great Verulam) sed inveniendum quid natura aut faciat aut ferat."[1] But after all, I am not certain that many of its failures may not have been owing to the want of skill or dexterity in the operator rather than inefficacy of the remedy. If the slow typhus you describe be really epidemic showing clear signs of contagion, an emetic on the 1st attack, agreeable to Lind[2] and other respectable writers, may sometimes, as in your own use, crop the disease in its bud. But this I apprehend depends on the contagion being received by the saliva and conveyed to the stomach. When rec^d by the cutaneous pores or inhaled in inspiration, as perhaps more often happens, it is too far out of the sphere of action of an emetic, and the disease accordingly runs its course. As we are but seldom able to trace the mode in which the morbid fomes is received into the body, I wou'd earnestly persuade a full and fair trial of the following method of prevention which has lately been found to counteract even the plague itself, not only as prophylactic but even cure when administered in the 1st stage of the disease. Let the patient be stripped in a warm room and powerfully rubbed with Oleum Oliva over the whole surface till copious perspiration ensues, which is to be encouraged in a warm bed and repeated evening and morn^g 3 or 4 times if need be, using near a pint of oil each operation. Let the diet be light, spoon meat of the vegetable kind and strict temperance observed. Let a journal of such cases be kept, and the genuine effects undisturbed by other remedies be noted, and then let me know the result. Dr Currie's tract on water in fevers etc. I have not seen.[3]—van Swieten and Morgagni I understood you have already read—after this, such volum^s writings, however excellent, are perhaps better calculated to refer to occasionally than to peruse again at so short a period, espec^y now that the theories of both are almost obsolete. I should rather advise writing cases imaginary, according to the classes of Sauvages or Cullen.[4] First simply, and next with complications, giving the prognosis, indications and ratio medendi, marking the contraindications. This I know to be highly useful to a young pract^r in preparing him for every case that may occur and giving him a promptitude and facility in prescribing not easily attainable by any other means. After this compare your practice with the best pract^l authors. While M^rs P[urlewent?] persists in leaving her case to chance 'tis but loss of time to suggest rational means. There is a duty belongs to the patient as well as the physic^n: both must conspire to effect a cure. With best wishes to Mrs Woodforde. Dr Sir

y^rs A. Fothergill

P.S. Your brother will I hope observe y^r instructions respecting the little arrear due to Dr Hawes which ought to be acknowledged as you rightly judge with gratitude.

[1] "One should not concoct or think out theoretically, but one should discover what nature does or brings". Francis Bacon (1561–1626), Viscount St Albans, Lord Verulam.

[2] James Lind (1716–1794), *Two papers on fevers and infection*, London, D. Wilson, 1763, pp. 59, 66.

[3] James Currie (1756–1805), *Medical reports, on the effects of water, cold and warm, as a remedy in fever, and febrile diseases . . . with observations on the nature of fever; and on the effects of opium, alcohol, and inanition*, Liverpool, M'Creery, for Cadell & Davies, London, 1797.

[4] One of many editions of François Boissier de Sauvages de la Croix (1706–1767), *Nosologia methodica, sistens morborum classes, juxta Sydenhami mentem et botanicorum ordinem*, Amsterdam, Bros de Tournes, 1763, and William Cullen, *Synopsis nosologiae methodicae*, Edinburgh, 1769. Subsequent editions were much revised.

N° 53 **58**

[no date or place][Bath,1798?][1]

My dear Sir,

Since y^r departure, I have been considering your dear mother's unfortunate case with attention and shall, agreeable to promise, briefly communicate the result. 1st It appears to me that the deafness, from whatever cause it might originate, is manifestly now connected with nervous debility, and relaxed tone of the tympanum. The secret^n of wax is prevented, and the Eustach^n tubes probably obstructed. The indications are to strengthen the nerv^s system in general—and the organ of hearing in particular—and to remove local obstruction. She must avoid tea, drastic or purg^g med^s, anxiety of mind or whatever weakens or enfeebles the system. On the contrary, she should use a generous diet, exercise in the open air, tonic remedies and sea bathing; the last in June and July. To excite the auditory nerves, and produce secretions of cerumen, brisk sternutat^s and electrical vibrations are perhaps the likeliest means that art can afford, as also towards removing obstructions in the Eustach^n tubes. To this end an injection thrown up the nostrils so as to pass thro' the tubes in the mouth deserves trial and likewise passed into the auditory passage. As she hears best during a loud noise she sh^d frequent the belfry when the bells are ringing a full peal, and habituate herself to this often, or to any other loud noise, as the report of fire arms or artillery. Lastly let her try at Evills the effect of the different hearing trumpets or acoustic machines, and keep one by her. With best wishes for her relief. I am, Dr Sir, on all occasions, y^rs very sincerely

A. Fothergill

[1] The reference to Woodforde's mother and her illness dates this letter.

N° 63 **59**

Bath Sep 28 1798

Dr Sir

Herewith I hope you'll receive safe Dr Currie and with thanks for the perusal, also the little pieces w^h I here inclose for y^r amusement and information. Dr Currie's method is a bold one and demands no small circumspection in those who may be induced to imitate it, since one unfortunate case may bring the pract^r the imputation of murder—such is the force of prejudice. I was no less struck with y^r adventurous scheme of translating Haller's Elementa Physiologiae, opus quidem arduum!![1] an undertaking w^h, like the conquest of Troy, wou'd require a ten year seige! Of all the Latin writers Haller is perhaps the most difficult, a studied obscurity pervades the work and however this might ans^r his intention of impressing it on the memory of his juvenile readers, it is presumed few will like to imitate it or to take it for a model. To translate the great work wou'd require the abilities of a 1st rate classic [scholar] and a through acquaintance with the German phraseology and the author's peculiar, abstruse mode of expression. These and other considerations have hitherto deterred English readers from any attempt of this sort. I cannot therefore advise you to such an irksome, unpromising undertaking. If you can read him so as to comprehend the main scope of his reasoning, be content with that. But if you want to improve your Latinity and attain an easy, perspicuous style take Boerhaave or van Swieten. I have just received a polite letter from His Excellency Count Berchtold who intends to translate my late tracts and disperse them thro' Italy and Germany.[2] His preservative and curative method in the plague will I trust save many lives and prove also efficac^s against typhus and yellow fever.[3] He recommends oleum oliva also against hydrophobia, and approves highly of what I hinted on that subject.

With best respects to Mrs Woodforde I remain

Dr Sir, much yours A. Fothergill

N.B. The new discovery of Galvani on the influence of metallic conductors in exciting nervous electricity[4] tends to confirm my theory and bids fair to be useful in many painful diseases espec^{y} such as are seated in the external muscles.

1 "A work which is indeed hard going".

2 Leopold von Berchtold (1750–1809) apparently did not do so.

3 Leopold von Berchtold, *Descrizione del nuovo rimedio curativo e preservativo contro la peste*, Vienna, F. A. Schraembl, 1797.

4 Luigi Galvani (1737–1798), *De viribus electricitatis in motu musculari commentarius, cum J. Aldini dissertatione et notis. Acc. epistolae ad animalis electricitatis theoriam pertinentes*, Modena, Soc. Typog., 1792.

N° 59 **60**

Bath 8^{ber} 16/98 [16 October 1798]

Dr Sir,

In your last letter are many passages over w^{h} I pored a long time without being able to decipher them. Mr Dawson who happen'd to be by was still more puzzled. I am therefore at a loss how to answer them.

I called at Cruttwells[1] on Sat^{y} and paid the cash to the assignees as you'll see from the enclosed receipt.

If you'll condense M^{rs} P[urlewent's?] case into a compact form and in a fair legible hand and send it to me I will transmit it to the editor of Med^{l} Facts[2] etc. Dr Reid's 2nd edit^{n}[3] I have not seen. The scrophul^{s} phthysis constitutes but one species and that no doubt is often hereditary. The heat after meals is rather owing to fresh chyle entering the vessels and passing thro' diseased lungs. Phlogiston is now a non-entity with the ablest chemists, and can be well spared from pathology. That the bronchæ abound in mucous glands cannot be denied, tho' chiefly not of the conglobate but conglomerate kind. The phlegm acquires thickness and viscosity from absorption of the aqueous part. The sebaceous glands secrete a different matter of an unctuous nature and are often enlarged and suppurate where there is no scrophula or hectic tendency. The primary cause of obstruction in both appears not to be inflammation but atonia. The suspension of hectic [fever] in mania seems rather owing to the deep mental impression w^{h} occupies the brain, and lessens determination to the lungs rather than diminution of blood or oxygen. Abscesses no doubt cause hectic symptoms in other organs as well as the lungs—but temperament and idiosyncrasy vary the symptoms.

Dr Reid's practice is rational, only too fond of emetics. Myrrh is by no means inert, but perhaps the main ingred^{t} in Griffith's mixture[4] but the whole is overrated and often misapplied. Neither Blane[5] nor Rush[6] have I yet seen. Currie's practice is sufficiently bold and may, without great care, bring a young practitioner into great disgrace. It is, however, ingenious and bespeaks a philosophical turn. From your letter it does not appear that you received my packet by the carrier the former week with w^{h} I returned Currie[7] with thanks and sent Falconer on diet[8] with some other small tracts for y^{r} entertainment, tho' doubtless he would take care to bring them from the full moon, not doubting this I did not ask him on Saturday last. According to your request of a French author I here send you to peruse M. Le Begue[9] of w^h you'll please to take great care being a very scarce book and not easy to be obtained.

A spare copy of my last ed^n on Cheltenham waters having cast up, it is at y^r service—so you need not return it. I believe now nothing of importance in your letter has escaped me. To comprehend the general meaning of Haller is one thing. To translate him correctly another. Beware of too intense study.

"Neque semper arcum tendit Apollo."[10]

with remembrance to Mrs Woodforde. Dr Sir

much y^rs A. Fothergill

[1] Probably R. Cruttwell of Bath, the publisher of Fothergill's tracts.

[2] The editor of *Medical facts* was Samuel Foart Simmons (1750–1813), physician, doctor of physic (Leyden 1776), FRS, licentiate of the College of Physicians (1778). In 1781, Simmons became the editor of *The London medical journal*, which issued a volume yearly from 1780 to 1790. The journal then changed its title to *Medical facts and observations* and Simmons remained as editor. Eight volumes of *Medical facts* were published between 1791 and 1800. Woodforde's account of Mrs. Purlewent's case was never published.

[3] Presumably, Thomas Reid, *An essay on the nature and cure of the phthisis pulmonalis. The second edition enlarged. To which is added an appendix on the use and effects of frequent vomits*, 2nd ed., London, T. Cadel [*sic*], 1785. First edition, 1782.

[4] Possibly Moses Griffith (1724–1785), physician, MD (Leyden 1744), London practitioner, credited with the invention of a "compound iron mixture of the Pharmacopoeia". William Munk, *The roll of the Royal College of Physicians*, 2nd ed., London, The College, 1878, vol. 2, pp. 164–5.

[5] Gilbert Blane (1749–1834), *Observations on the diseases incident to seamen*, London, printed by J. Couper & sold by J. Murray, 1785; third edition, London, Murray & Highley, 1799.

[6] Benjamin Rush (1745–1813), *Medical inquiries and observations*, 5 vols., Philadelphia, T. Dobson, 1794–98.

[7] See letter **59**.

[8] William Falconer (1744–1824), *Observations on some of the articles of diet and regimen usually recommended to valetudinarians*, London, 1778.

[9] Possibly, Achille-Guillaume Le Bègue de Presle (1735?–1807), *Le conservateur de la santé, ou avis sur les dangers qu'il importe à chacun d'éviter, pour se conserver en bonne santé et prolonger sa vie. On y a joint des objets de reglemens de police relatifs à la santé*, Paris, P. F. Didot, Jnr., 1763.

[10] "Nor does Apollo always bend his bow". Horace, *Odes*, 2.10.19–20. See also letter **9**.

N° 61 **61**

Bath Nov: 3/98

Accept, Dear Sir, my best thanks for your obliging present of a fine pheasant; I am glad to hear my 2 packets reached you safe. Y^r affecting account of y^r dear mother's relapse into such a deplorable state of debility gives me great concern. I have considered y^r account with much attention and happy indeed should I be cou'd I suggest any thing that might add efficacy to the measures you have already so judiciously pursued, or ward off for sometime longer an event w^h you see just cause to deprecate. If this be not an entire breaking up of constitution, somewhat still perhaps may be done for her relief, especially as you are constantly with her. At all events y^r tender care and attention in addition to y^r professional skill afford her no common consolation. On the next page I shall sketch out the heads of the treatment w^h appear to me advisable, w^h you can vary as circumstances point out. In addition to w[h] I sh[d] recommend both upper and lower extremities and the course of the spine to be powerfully rubbed every even[g] till a general glow or perspiration ensue, with camphorated oil, wearing flannel next the skin. With the close of the medical journal I dropped the work and have only seen the 1st vol. of Med[l] Facts, so know nothing when the 8th will appear, tho' most likely in the usual course.[1] Agreeable to y[r] request I shall look over the case with pen in hand and write to D[r] Simmons,[2] but think you must allow him to abridge it, sh[d] he be scarce of room, in such an extensive correspondence from all quarters. As I cannot have the pleasure of y[r] company to partake of the bird here, I think it will be acceptable in London and shall therefore accompany the packet this even[g] by the mail. That you may have the supreme satisfaction of administering relief to y[r] afflicted parent is the fervent wish of, D[r] Sir, y[rs] ever A. Fothergill

[1] The transcription is 1st but 7th would make more sense. But Fothergill iterates 1st in the next letter where it does make sense, and in Letter **74** he asks for the 2nd and subsequent volumes. *The London medical journal* closed in 1790. The first volume of *Medical facts and observations* appeared in 1791 and the seventh in 1797 but the eighth and last appeared in 1800.

[2] Samuel Foart Simmons, see letter **60**, note 2.

N[o] 64 **62**

Bath Feb 16/1799

D[r] Sir,

Tho' much pressed for time, I instantly ans[r] y[r] lett[r] to be in time for the carr[rs] return, for certainly not a moment ought to be lost. That a congestion is going on in the cavities of the brain seems highly probable, however that nothing may be wanting in this truly deplorable case that may contribute to y[r] mother's relief, or the satisfaction of y[r] self or friends I think (so far as can be judged at this distance) it will be advisable to proceed as follows on the subsequent page.

In consequence of the floods, travelling is almost impracticable as I experienced yest[y] in the neighbourhood of Frome. The same difficulty prevails abroad. No mails due to F[h] embargo. D[r] Lowder[1] a few days ago requested a perusal of M[c]bride otherwise it wou'd accompany the lett[r]. Having dropped Duncan's Comments[2] and also the Med[l] Journal[3] when it changed its title and order of publication and only seen the 1st vol. of Med[l] Facts etc. I cou'd wish to see the remaining vols. with y[r] next letter, for I shall be impatient to hear how y[r] poor mother is, and whether it be within the compass to ward off the impending blow. To disburden the brain is the manifest intention but I fear she is too feeble to bear drastic purges—safer perhaps by stimulating clysters. Let the head be elevated and the feet kept warm, perhaps mild sinapisms[4] might be useful. With best wishes I remain D[r] Sir in extreme haste y[rs] assuredly

A. Fothergill

[1] Possibly William Lowder (1740–1801), MD (Aberdeen 1775), Licentiate of RCP (1786).

[2] Andrew Duncan, the elder, editor of *Medical and philosophical commentaries by a society of physicians in Edinburgh*. Twenty volumes of the journal appeared between 1773 and 1795. From 1796 to 1804, the journal was continued as *Annals of medicine*, also published in Edinburgh.
[3] *The London medical journal* changed its title to *Medical facts and observations* in 1791.
[4] Mustard poultices.

N° 57 **63**

[no date or place][February 1799?][1]

D[r] Sir

The late inundations retarded my last as they have also the post in various places. On Thursday last I rode deep in water and was afterwards caught in the severe storm of wind rain thunder and lightning, since w[h] I have been feverish and much indisposed. Your packet this morning came safe but I was out and had not a moment of time to ans[r] y[r] very satisfactory letter till now, so must send per post. As the med[s] proposed have warded off the fatal stroke longer than we had reason to expect we shall not cease, while life remains, to use every effort to keep the machine in motion, as it must give you future satisfaction to reflect that nothing essential has been omitted. The extravasated fluid compresses the brain in various parts but particularly about the origin of the optic nerves, hence the loss of vision. Hence too the turgescency of the face with heat, flushing and febrile pulse. The brain has few lymphat[s] and absorption there is tardy even in young subjects, so that we have every difficulty to struggle with. The sympt[s] seem to warrant further depletion, as the only chance. Abstinence too sh[d] be used as a main auxiliary, and perhaps wine had better be omitted, as we must study to keep down the symptom[l] fever and keep the system as cool and temperate as possible. With best wishes for her relief, I am, D[r] Sir, yours sincerely

A. Fothergill

P.S. Should she still be alive when this reaches you, proceed as follows as circumstances shall point out.

[1] The floods (see letter **62**) and the reference to Woodforde's sick mother roughly date this letter. The weather was very severe in February 1799. *Gentleman's Magazine*, 1799, **69**: pt. 1, 246.

N° 58 **64**

[no date or place][1799][1]

D[r] Sir,

This day I was fav[d] with your obliging letter but not till the post had set out. Having hitherto warded off the final stroke longer than cou'd have been reasonably expected, we must still strive to diminish the congestion in the encephalon which perverts the functions of the brain, and w^h supports the disease in its original character. I cannot help suspecting from y^r last acc^t that she takes more food and that too of the animal kind than is consistent with the plan of depletion. "Quo magis nutriveris (says Hippocrates in such cases) eo magis laedit."[2] In such cases of an oppressed brain, food will not nourish, nor tonics afford strength. Arteriotomy surpasses cupping or venesection as it removes at once a quantity of arterial blood, and should therefore still have a trial as far as [10 or 12 Apothecary ounces].[3] The digitalis, remarkable for diminishing the velocity of the pulse and producing a copious flow of urine, should at least once a day receive a fuller a trial. I think I mentioned a sternutatory with Pulv: Asari with a little Elleb: Alb:[4] which from your silence does not appear to have been used. On mature deliberation respecting this critical situation I think in addit^n to abstemious diet the following should be the outlines of the present treatment. I feel for her sufferings and am Dr Sir yours assuredly

A. Fothergill

[1] The worsening sickness of Woodforde's mother dates this to spring 1799.

[2] "The more you feed, the more harm it does". Hippocrates, *Aphorisms*, vii, 68. The particular Latin translation of the original Greek has not been identified.

[3] Fothergill gave the prescription in Apothecary signs.

[4] Pulvis Asari was made from the leaves of Asarabacca. Elleborus Albus was one of the names for white hellebore.

N° 60 **65**

Bath June 14/99

Dear Sir,

Nothing but time, I well know, can restore tranquility to a mind suffering the pangs of grief for the loss of an affectionate parent. Letters of common condolence serve but to renew the affliction and are therefore ill-judged and impertinent. This, I trust, will sufficiently apologize for my late silence. The mind must have still longer time to recover its tone and before that aching void you yet experience can be completely removed. It was not without surprise that I rec^d your last dated from Crewkerne, especially as you had repeatedly expressed y^r satisfaction in being so prosperously established in y^r native soil, and so well content with the prospect of increasing practice. The step you have taken is a bold one, and it is hoped those friends who have advised it will make a point of contributing to y^r establishment, and prevent the necessity of an unpleasant retrograde retreat to Castle Cary among old friends with perhaps new faces. At Castle Cary you had no competition, at Crewkerne you have already 2 and will have to scramble for one third of the booty among strangers. Besides you know the old proverb tho' I hope you may prove an exception to the general result. Lyme cannot but have at least 1 resident physi^n every summer, and therefore not to be depended upon. Patients from hence go to Southampton and Weymouth not to Lyme, at least very few. From Dr Daniel[1] I once had a letter or two but no other correspondence or interview. If his practice ever amounted to 700^£ or even 600, it exceeded considerably what I sh^d conceive, and am clear that these calculations are generally exaggerated, of w[h] we had a late instance at Bath. In such times as these when every little town is overstocked, and apoth[s] engross almost the whole business, it will behove physicians to moderate their expectations and live very oeconomically. Wishing you that degree of success as may be most conducive to y[r] happiness. I remain

D[r] Sir, y[rs] assuredly
A. Fothergill

P.S. The Med[l] Facts I have not till just now had time to dip into, but shall skim over them at leisure and then inquire some mode of safe conveyance.

[1] Presumably Samuel Daniel (1755?–1798?), MD (Edinburgh 1776), extra-Licentiate of the College of Physicians (1777), practised in Crewkerne, Somerset.

N[o] 66 **66**

Bath 7[ber] 30/99 [30 September 1799]

Y[r] last very obliging letter, my dear sir, claims my early acknowledgement. The perusal of such lett[rs] breathing the warm effusions of friendship recalls a thousand pleasing ideas and presents to the mind, after many years have elapsed, a scene of renewed gratification and entertainment. Select lett[rs] of this kind, I have always carefully treasured up, and cou'd not, without doing violence to my feelings, commit entire bundles of lett[rs] indiscriminately (as some do) to the flames. Some indeed it wou'd be wrong to preserve—others it wou'd be a kind of sacrilege to destroy. Partiality to our friends ought not to prevent us from making the necessary discrimination, tho' I must confess it often disposes me to lean to the favorable side and I am not sorry to find it inclines you to the same bias. It however carries you to excess when you talk of transcribing my letters, and reading them in conjunction with D[r] Gregory's excellent work on Duties of a Physician!

Friendship, peculiar boon of Heav'n,
The noble mind's delight and pride,
To men and Angels only giv'n,
To all the lower world denied,[1]

Friendship, however, like love, sometimes hoodwinks the judgement. It therefore behoves the philosopher to guard against the excesses of both.

But now ad rem—time presses! I am sorry I have not the authors on the materia medica you mention or they sh[d] accomp[y] this. M[c]bride it seems you have got nearer home and I here send you by the Weymouth coach, Hippocrates 2 tom[s], a curious memoir on the mammoth's bones from a learned judge of the western territory,[2] and my copy on rabies canina just published.[3] With the packet you mention please to return the French tract on corrosive sublimate and Dr Gibbes's Syllabus of Chem[y4] etc. In revising M.S. and other engagements have not had time to skim over y[r] med[l] journals, but will return on short notice if wanted. D[r] Sir, y[rs] assuredly

A. Fothergill

[1] Samuel Johnson, *Friendship: an ode*.

[2] We have been unable to trace this reference. References to the early literature on mammoths is to be found in Rembrandt Peale, *Account of the skeleton of the mammoth, a non-descript carnivorous animal of immense size*, London, E. Lawrence, 1802. See letter **85** where Fothergill meets the creature face to face.

[3] Anthony Fothergill, *An essay on the nature of the disease occasioned by the bite of a mad dog*, Bath, 1799.

[4] George Smith Gibbes (1771–1851), *Syllabus of a course of chemical lectures*, Bath, W. Meyler, 1799.

N° 56 **67**

Bath Sat: 9 Nov 99

Dear Sir

Herewith you'll receive warm from the press, tho' somewhat disfigured with corrections, my new essay, being the 1st copy that has seen the light, being as yet not published.[1] With it I return with thanks y^{r} 6 vols. of med^{l} tracts extending to the begin^{g} of 1797, f^{m} w^{h} period to the close of the present year 2 more vols. must I think be in readiness for the subscribers.[2] The omission of the prices of books is a capital defect as I long ago hinted to the author but it still remains, and an almost useless catalogue swells the vol. and adds to the expense —the long winded cases in surgery in particular want the pruning knife, still, however, the work is a useful one, only too prolix. Before our Philosophical Soc^{y} last night I read a long interesting letter with w^{h} I was lately fav^{d} by an ingenious Philadelphian[3] on a new remedy against dysentery and lues venerea. Also on origin and prevention of the pestilential fever, which you may see when you come next to Bath.

Bradley and Willich's medical magazine,[4] it seems, increases in reputation and in orig^{l} papers. The new Analyt: Review defunct.[5] I hope you rec^{d} safe 1 Oct. by Weymouth coach: Hippocrates opera, 2 tomes, Essay on mammoth, and my copy (for revision) on rabies canina.[6] The former parcel sent Feb. 18—tract on corrosive sublimate, Gibbes's Chemical Syllabus, woods poor bill[7] etc. it is presumed you have done with long ago. Some of the books a phys^{n} here wishes to see, but if you have looked over the passages you wished to see in Hippocrates he must wait a little till you return the whole in one parcel by the carrier, for the Weymouth coach is I think stopped for the winter. Dr Haygarth on the Tractors is in the press[8] w^{h} I hope to have when published as you need not buy it.

Dr Sir, much yours. A. Fothergill

P.S. My boy sends the enclosed to his mother.

[1] Probably Anthony Fothergill, *An essay on the preservation of shipwrecked mariners*, London, 1799. Fothergill had already sent his work on rabies, published the same year. See letter **66**, note 4.

[2] Eight volumes of *Medical facts and observations* were published, the last in 1800.

[3] Presumably Benjamin Rush, the Philadelphian physician.

[4] Anthony Florian Madinger Willich (?–?) and Thomas Bradley (1751–1813) were editors of *The medical and physical journal*, which first appeared in March 1799.

[5] *The analytical review; or history of literature domestic and foreign, etc*, (May 1788–December 1798), 28 vols., London, 1788–99.

[6] See letter **66**, note 3.

[7] Reference unclear.

[8] John Haygarth (1740–1827), *Of the imagination, as a cause and as a cure of disorders of the body; exemplified by fictitious tractors, and epidemical convulsions. Read to the Literary and Philosophical Society*

of Bath, Bath, R. Cruttwell, 1800. Haygarth was a distinguished physician living in Bath at 15 Royal Crescent from 1798. Fothergill, however, makes no personal references to him. See Introduction, p. xxii.

N° 67 **68**

Bath Decr 28^{h}/99

Many thanks D^{r} D^{r}, for your kind and seasonable present of a very fine turkey of w^{h}, as I cannot hope for the pleasure of y^{r} comp^{y}, to partake next week with a few friends we shall drink y^{r} health with three cheers. You are right and I was wrong, I had overlooked the French tract w^{h} had fallen behind other books. In return for y^{r} kindness and my own remissness please to accept these little tracts w^{h} are much at y^{r} service. The case you relate is remarkable and the event must be extremely doubtful. The symp^{s} seem evidently to proceed f^{m} injury of the spinal marrow—whether this be irreparable will depend on the degree of injury and the patient's fate will probably be determined within a few days. The brach^{l} nerves seem to have suffered more than those of the lower extremities hence their motion more difficult to restore, but this happens also in palsies from an internal cause. A copious discharge from the lower part of the nape of the neck will give the best chance, but beware of removing too much blood or enfeebling the system. Slight electr^{l} shocks along the course of the spine may prove beneficial, and keeping up a free perspiration with guaiacum. Time presses and, the carrier ready to set off, must therefore here drop the pen, but not without best wishes for y^{r} health and success thro' many happy returns of the season—Dear Sir

much yours adieu!

<u>A. Fothergill</u>

N° 65 **69**

Bath Frid: Night /2 past 12 O'clock [January 1800?]

Y^{r} lett^{r}, D^{r} D^{r}, dated the 8th came this afternoon in my absence, as I find it now on my return past midnight. Nevertheless as the case is truly urgent I snatch up the pen at this late hour to ans^{r} it without delay. I have considered with attention your accurate and circumstantial acc^{t}, and do sincerely sympathize with you on the young woman's case. The main symp^{ts}, as you justly observe, give strong suspicion of internal dropsy of the brain, yet so far as I can judge at this distance they afford only presence of water in the cavities of that organ. The <u>adult age</u>, the <u>absence of dilation</u> of the pupils, of <u>strabismus</u> and of <u>convulsions</u>, all dispose me to hope the case may not be so wholly desperate. That there is, however, a preternatural determination of blood to the encephalon is, I think highly probable, and that there may also be irritation in the primæ viæ from worms of larger size, w^{h} may render the case more complex and more equivocal. Sh^{d} the above symptoms however appear y^{r}

mercurial plan will give perhaps the best chance. On the next page I shall put down what seems to be the ratio medendi but must leave it to be modified by you who are on the spot, and watch with anxiety the progress of the disease. At all events the long abst^{d} calam: [?] the plethoric habit, and determinat^{ns} to the brain demands active evacuants. That nature may second y^{r} endeavours and y^{t} you may have the comfort of restoring this young woman is the sincere wish D^{r} D^{r}, y^{rs} affectionately

P.S. Y^{r} fine turkey on {A. Fothergill

Monday last proved exquisite, and helped to regale a select party of a dozen friends among whom I wished for y^{r} presence. PS: Your prudent practical plan of study I much commend.

N° 72 **70**

Bath Aug: 23. 1800

Dear Sir,

My late London journey w^{h} took up a whole week deprived me of the pleasure of seeing you as well as 2 other med^{l} gentlemen who came here on urgent business during my absence, as did also Dr Renaudet on a visit the day before I set out, whom I was very sorry to leave. Such cross incidents are to be regretted but can neither be foreseen or prevented. Your obliging letter of yesterday (tho' much pressed for time) I must now briefly ans^{r} as the carrier is ready to return. Marcard's performance[1] I have not read, but am not quite satisfied with the term tonic as applied to the tepid bath. Anodyne sedative emollient wou'd have been more appropriate, much less can I approve of Darwin's[2] advice of a bath at the temperature of 96 to 98 for half an hour every day. Such unqualified assertions tend to mislead young practitioners. Both extremes of hot and cold bathing are too indiscriminately used and are productive of many serious evils under the present empirical practice, the result of ignorance and fashionable caprice. In country practice where a warm bath is required the elegancy and conveniency of our baths here cannot be expected or obtained, but a narrow bathing tub or semicubrium ought to be had in every market town. A tin one invented at Manchester and called a Couchett [?] may be had of any capital tin man in Lond^{n} but the price I suppose is pretty high. The tin shower bath is common, but a very imperfect contrivance. The digitalis indeed retards the velocity of the pulse and seems to me to suspend, but by no means cure a hectic fever, and the extreme debility and cold sweats induced, I fear, often more than counterbalance its supposed specific power on the heart and arterial system. Without extreme caution and good manag^{t} it may often tend to precipitate an event we wish to retard. This is not meant to discourage prudent trials, but to impress caution. "Valeat itaq quod valere potest."[3] Wine no doubt may be advantageously used. Clysters arise where indurated[?], or deglutition interrupted. Cold liquids may be given in typhus, tho' few prudent practitioners will presume to plunge the sick (as some advise) into a cold bath. The pain or rather anxiety in hydrothorax is rather f^{m} pressure on the diaphragm and mediastinum than on the stomach or liver.

Thornton's second edit^{n},[4] Burserius[5] and Duncan's Hoff^{n}[6] I have not seen. In haste, D^{r} D^{r} I remain much yours. A. Fothergill

[1] Heinrich Matthias Marcard (1747–1817), *A short description of Pyrmont*, London, 1788.
[2] Probably Erasmus Darwin. Source not found.
[3] "So let that be strong which can be strong". Not attributable.
[4] Presumably, Robert John Thornton (1768?–1837), *Medical extracts: on the nature of health. New edition*, London, Robinson, etc., 1794. New edition, London, J. Johnson, 1796–97.
[5] Presumably, Giovanni Battista Borsieri (1725–1785), *Institutionum medicinae practicae, quas auditoribus suis praelegebat J. B. Burserius*, 4 vols., Milan, 'Typ. Imp. Mon. S. Ambrosii Majoris', 1781–89; or, *The institutions of the practice of medicine . . . Translated from the Latin by William Cullen Brown*, 1 vol., Edinburgh, W. Mudie, 1800.
[6] Friedrich Hoffmann, *A system of the practice of medicine; from the Latin. . . . [Translated] By . . . W. Lewis. . . . Revised . . . by A. Duncan*, 2 vols., London, J. Murray & J. Johnson, 1783.

N° 71 **71**

Bath 9^{ber} [November] 1800

Dear Sir,

Your accurate description of Mr Hall's case (whom you obligingly recommended to my care) I have maturely considered, together with all the phenomena the disease presents to us on close examination. The severity of the pain has from time to time been alleviated and the cure, by the suitable means employed, wou'd probably have been effected some time ago, had not the obstruction been uncommonly stubborn, whether invincible, time will discover. That the ductus communis,[1] tho' not entirely, yet remains in a great measure blocked up is evident, and most probably from biliary concretions of the rugged angular kind, w^{h} however we may hope, in time, to dislodge and that all may do well, provided that the organic structure of the liver be not irreparably injured, particularly the posterior part of the lobe w^{h} eludes the touch.[2] In w^{h} case the adjacent pancreas generally partakes of the affection. At present I have the satisfaction to acquaint you that the Bath water both internally and exter^{y} agrees well, and that the pain is less frequent and less intense as the disease produces torpor. I wish much to discontinue opium as much as may be, f^{m} w^{h} nothing can be expected beyond that of a palliative. As such however may sometimes be indispensable. If the jaundice continue much longer it will probably end in a confirmed dropsy, of w^{h} the oedema of the ankles seems to be the harbinger. In short, the case is beset with many unpromising circumstances, to w^{h} the season of the year and very humid atmosphere will add, I fear, insurmountable difficulties. The angina scarlatina[3] with a dark bloated appearance of the tonsils has of late made its attack on several persons, partic^{y} the weak and relaxed, of w^{h}, f^{m} the pressure of the times, and scarce and bad provisions, we see too many instances. Such predisposing causes, in my opinion, militate strongly against bleeding, or other enfeebling evacuations.[4] The buffy surface of the blood is too apt to impose us in this and many other cases of malignancy of w^{h} the scarlet efflorescence is a mark in the above cases. Whether the cynanche trachealis or croup was not complicated with the scarlatina in the 2 unhappy boys you mention, I am not quite clear, tho' I suspect it. You add the sister and the father also fell victims (dreadful fatality) but afterwards you say both escaped—how can this be? But your letter seems written in such haste, I cannot make out many passages. The season modifies the disease and causes it sometimes to exhibit sloughs, often not, as in the present case, tho' perhaps more highly dangerous than when accompanied with ash color'd specks, even deep ulcers of the tonsils only, but the danger increases in proportion as the larynx suffers. The genuine croup seems confined to child^{n} f^{m} 3 to 12 or 14 and is known by the peculiar sound of the voice like that of a young cock attempting to crow. No scarlet erruptions, no tumified tonsils—the tracheal sloughy membrane not the cause but consequence. The disease not yet proved to be contagious. Hence you'll see it differs in its essence from angina scarlatina. To cure the former we must prevent the formation of the membrane w^{h} is an exudation of the albumen of the blood. A work of no small difficulty, but w^{h} may be accomplished if we can render absorption equal or superior to the exhalation. Of this and other topics more when we meet. Meanwhile I remain, D^{r} D^{r} yours

assuredly
A. Fothergill

[1] The common bile duct.

[2] Here, as in letter **54**, is evidence of the physical examination of patients.

[3] Fevers, with severe throat, notably angina scarlatina and croup, were the subject of much nosographic interest in the eighteenth century, notably among authors writing in English. See John Fothergill, *An account of the sore throat attended with ulcers*, London, C. Davis, 1748; John Huxham (1692–1768), *A dissertation on the malignant, ulcerous, sore throat*, London, J. Hinton, 1757; Francis Home, *An enquiry into the nature, cause, and cure of the croup*, Edinburgh, A. Kincaid & J. Bell, 1765; Samuel Bard (1742–1821), *An enquiry into the nature, cause and cure, of the angina suffocativa*, New York, S. Inslee & A. Car, 1771. Later authors have identified these descriptions with either scarlet fever or diphtheria.

[4] John Fothergill, whom Anthony much admired (see Introduction, pp. xi–xii, and Letter **1**) opposed bleeding in this condition. "How many lives were lost", wrote William Withering in 1793, "until Dr Fothergill and Dr Wall taught us to withold the lancet and the purge". Cited in R. H. Fox, *Dr John Fothergill and his friends*, London, Macmillan, 1919, p. 54.

N° 68 **72**

Bath Dec^{r}: 17, 1800

Dear Sir

Amidst a variety of letters w^{h} demand prompt dispatch, I have time to acknowledge y^{r} obliging present of a fine hare, and to pack up for y^{r} perusal Hewson's 2 vols. on Lymph^{s} and Opera Sydenham,[1] the only ones I can lay my hands on at present the rest being invisible—part lent and part perhaps exchanged for others, especially Baglivi.[2] Those forwarded will however be sufficient, I presume, to occupy all y^{r} spare time if you go carefully thro' them before we meet. Till then D^{r} D^{r} adieu

Dreadful times! A. Fothergill

Bella, bella! horrida bella![3]

[1] Presumably one of the many editions of Thomas Sydenham (1624–1689), *Opera universa . . . Editio altera, priori multum auctior, etc.*, 2 pts., London, R. N. for W. Kettilby, 1685.

[2] Possibly one of the many editions of Giorgio Baglivi (1668–1707), *Opera omnia medico-practica et anatomica*, Lyon, Annison & J. Posuel, 1704.

[3] "Wars! horrible wars!". Virgil, *Aeneid*, 6.86.

N° 69 **73**

[No place or date][1801?][1]

Dear Sir,

Y^{r} lett^{rs} written volante calamo[2] neither myself nor Mr Dawson, who happened to be with me, cou'd perfectly decipher, w^{h} inter nos will I hope be a caution to you in future, especially in letters of such consequence, where every iota ought to be perfectly legible. For it will not avail you who can write well to plead the example of some physicians whose half-formed letters or rather execrable hieroglyphics can never be made out but by guess, and w^{h} occasion very often, dangerous errors, to say nothing of the waste of time in hammering out the meaning. From what I can collect as to the present case, w^{h} I have considered with much attention, the symptoms seem to proceed f^{m} indigestion and an impaired tone of the alimentary canal. Hence the flatulency, eructations and disordered motion of the heart and arterial system, impaired vision, vertigo etc. This affection I imagine has been coming on more than a month ago, and if you inquire more minutely into his history, constitutional habit, mode of life, etc. (concerning w^{h} you are silent) you'll be able to trace the malady to some error in eating, drinking, semin^{l} evacuation, sedentary life etc., to w^{h} attention must be paid in the treatment. From this view of the case and connected, as it manifestly appears to be, with debility, there can be no room I conceive for bleeding or any large evacuation. But to judge with exactness at this distance, without seeing the patient is impossible, and particularly as to the propriety of sea bathing. Tho' y^{r} tonic plan seems eligible, yet where the digestive organs are weak, it cannot be too simple. If no material benefit result f^{m} a ten day trial of the following, a course of the Bath waters, the effic^{y} of w^{h} in dyspepsia is so well established, ought to be had recourse to.

I need not add that strict temperance must be enjoined "alias laterem tantum lavas."[3]

Sydenham arrived safe and has afforded you an excellent example of accurate observation, and elegant Latinity. Your med^{l} jourls, f^{m} incessant interruptions and large vol^{s} obtruded upon me to read and examine, I am sorry to say have been detained longer than intended, having yet not got thro' the 1st vol. but I hope now to proceed as fast as other avocations will allow. I have only room to add my best wishes for your success in your matrimonial[4] and all other laudable pursuits Dr Sir, adieu! A. Fothergill

[1] The reference to Woodforde's forthcoming marriage dates this as 1801. The reference to Sydenham seems to indicate situating the letter here. Accurate dating gets more difficult from here on.

[2] "With flying pen". See also letter **23**.

[3] "Otherwise you are just washing a brick". Not attributable. "Washing a brick" was proverbial for wasted effort.

[4] On Woodforde's marriage, see Introduction, p. xvii.

N° 70 **74**

Bath 7^{ber} [September] 25th 1800 [1801?][1]

Dear Sir,

Accept my thanks for your obliging letter and kind present w^{h} accompanied it. I am

pleased to hear your patient is better and that the theory thus far seems to be confirmed by the practice. As a slight error, however, in diet or regimen may readily renew the disorder, too great care cannot be taken to guard against a relapse, to remedy w^h^ will require no less than a course of Bath water drunk at the fountain head. Of your 3 vol^s^ of med^l^ journal I have looked over 1st and 2nd replete with multifarious observations, consisting, as we generally find in miscellaneous works of this kind, observations and remarks of very dissimilar merit.

"Quædam bona, quædam mala, mediocria quædam." [2]

The good however preponderate and render the work sufficiently interesting.

These vols. I return now with thanks, by the carrier and hope to finish the 3rd ere long and return it with Dr Lettsom's new publication on vaccination[3] expected daily and w^h^ you therefore need not buy. I am glad I have the 4 vols you wish to see of Whyte on nervous disorders[4] and 3 vols College Transactions[5]—w^h^ being books of frequent reference, please to keep clean and let me have them by the end of Octr and if by that time you can conveniently spare for a few weeks Duncan's Annals (or continuation of the Commentaries[6] from the end of the 20th vol., w^h^ 20 vols I have) and Simmons's Med^l^ Facts f^m^ 2 vol. down to the present time (w^h^ I understood him is to close the work) you'll oblige Dear D^r^

y^rs^ sincerely

A. Fothergill

P.S. Some new public^s^ are commended, but not yet with in these libraries, as Medical and Chirurgical Review,[7] Ferriar[8] and Rush's[9] Essays, Saunders on Min^l^ Waters,[10] Whately on Gonorrhea[11] and some Edin^r^ Med^l^ Theses, but the cowpox continues to absorb the attention of the med^l^ world beyond all other subjects.—Vale

[1] The reference to Lettsom, note 3 below, dates this as 1801.

[2] "Some things good, some things bad, some in-between". Not attributable.

[3] John Coakley Lettsom, *Observations on the cow-pock*, London, J. Mawman, 1801.

[4] Robert Whytt (1714–1766), *Observations on the nature, causes, and cure of those disorders which have commonly been called nervous, hypochondriac, or hysteric*, London, T. Becket and P. A. du. Hondt, 1765. The reference to 4 volumes is puzzling.

[5] *Medical transactions*, published by the Royal College of Physicians of London, London, vol. 1, 1768, vol. 2, 1772, vol. 3, 1785.

[6] Andrew Duncan, the elder, editor of *Annals of medicine*, Edinburgh, 1796–1804, the continuation of his *Medical and philosophical commentaries*, Edinburgh, 1773–95, vols. 1–20. See letter **62**.

[7] Presumably the journal, *The medical and chirurgical review*, London, begun in May 1794, ended January 1808.

[8] Possibly, John Ferriar (1761–1815), *Medical histories and reflections*, vol. 1, 1792, vol. 2, 1795, vol. 3, 1798, Warrington; London, printed by W. Eyres etc., for T. Cadell.

[9] Benjamin Rush, *Essays, literary, moral and philosophical*, Philadelphia, [printed by] T. & S. F. Bradford, 1798.

[10] William Saunders (1743–1817), *A treatise on the chemical history and medical powers of some of the most celebrated mineral waters*, London, W. Phillips, 1800.

[11] Thomas Whately (d. 1821), *Practical observations on the cure of the gonorrhoea virulenta in men*, London, J. Johnson, 1801.

N° 74 **75**

Bath Sat[y] 10[ber] [December] 26th [1801][1]

Dear Sir,

Herewith according to promise, I return with many thanks by M[r] Bennett all y[r] bound vols., No 8 [of *Medical facts*][2] and 1 N° of Phys[l] Journ[l] and consequently 4 N[os] of the journ[l] remain with me, w[h] I have not had time to glance over.[3] I also send for y[r] entertainment Dr Lettsom's new publication on vaccination,[4] an interesting work particularly to young Benedictines destined to produce a beautiful race of children, and therefore make no doubt y[r] amiable partner will also carefully peruse it as a matter of mutual concern. I also send D[r] Falconer's new tract on prevention of the plague[5] etc, w[h] I have only just received but not read—you may keep both, however, till towards the end of January when I hope to return the 4 N° of Phys[l] Journ[l]. I regretted y[r] stay here was so short, but hope you had a safe if not pleasant journey home. Bath is still by no means so full as was expected and what adds to the gloom the rainy season presents to constant view, cloud caped hills and muddy streets w[h] keep our belles and beaux in close winter quarters and ushers in the Xmas festival under sombre aspect. The definitive treaty however, now anxiously expected will, it is hoped, when it arrives brighten the scene, and peace attended with the loves and graces once more rekindle joy in every countenance. Then will all the nations of Europe have cause to rejoice and having weathered out the horrors of war look forward with complacency to better days and a more genial season.

"Aspice venturo laetentur ut omnia saeclo."[6]

That you and M[rs] Woodforde may live happy and see many such seasons is the fervent wish of,
Dear Sir,

yours assuredly

A. Fothergill

[1] This dating is tentative, the evidence for 1801 is: December 26 was a Saturday in 1801; Lettsom's work referred to as "new" appeared in 1801; the promise to return volumes of the *Medical and physical journal* in February was carried out in 1802. The reference to a definitive treaty would seem to suggest the Treaty of Amiens, 25 March 1802 (a preliminary peace agreement was signed in 1801). However the reference to Falconer on plague, published in 1802, creates problems unless it was published at the end of 1801 and carried the following year's imprint, a not unusual practice.

[2] See letters **61** and **74**. Volume 8 which appeared in 1800 was the last in the series.

[3] *The medical and physical journa*l, London, 1799–1814. Published 2 vols. per year beginning in March 1799. Six volumes should have appeared by the date of this letter, and it seems Woodforde still had volume 6 in his keeping. See letter **76**.

[4] See letter **74**.

[5] William Falconer, *Examination of Dr. Heberden's observations on the increase and decrease of different diseases, particularly the plague*, Bath, 1802. Also note, William Heberden, the younger (1767–1845), *Observations on the increase and decrease of different diseases and particularly of the plague*, London, 1801.

[6] "See how all things rejoice in the age/century that is to come". Virgil, *Eclogues*, 4.52.

N° 79 **76**

Bath Feb 24th 1802

Dr Sir,

Mr D.—the unfortunate young gentleman whose case you accurately describe and whom you properly recommended to try a course of these salutary waters under my care, I have the pleasure to inform you appears to be in a progressive way of amendment. The water agrees well and begins to shew restorative effects, but a case of this nature, the most obstinate and perhaps difficult to treat with propriety of any in the whole circle of practice, demands every additional resource and attention to the mental as well as corporeal faculties and withall a longer course than I fear his time will allow. But more of this in my next. The youth you mention who labours under petechiæ sine febre, will I make no doubt do well under the judicious regimen you advise. From the late scarcity and bad provisions, the blood has been impoverished and the solids deprived of due tone, no wonder that cases of this kind are more frequent than formerly and more tedious in the cure. In addition to the remedies you have so properly ordered, I wou'd recommend (should similar cases occur) nitrs acid and spruce beer for common beverage because the former readily evolves oxygen, the latter carbonic gas both of wh are peculiarly indicated.[1] The 2 tracts I lent you came safe by Mr D[awson?]—and I am glad they afforded you and Mrs Woodforde useful information.

The remaining 4 numbers of Medl and Physil Journal[2] wh you kindly sent for my inspection I perused with much satisfaction and have committed them to the care of Mr D[awson?]—who undertakes to forward them safely by the family now about to return home. As the 6th No[3] did not appear I suppose you had begun to read and had not got thro' it, or it wou'd have accompanied the other five. Their correspondence seems very extensive and the work abounds with original papers of different degrees of merit as must be expected. "Quædam bona, quædam mala, mediocria quædam."[4] But, all in all it is a work no young practitioner shd be without. Dr Simmons's London Medl Journal and also his subsequent tracts and observations are, I suppose, wholly discontinued.

Whether Duncan's Commentaries (wh I went on with to the end of the 20th vol.)[5] be continued with its wonted care in selections and former popularity I know not. You can perhaps tell if you continue the work. The state of medicine at Edinr as well as on the continent used to afford interesting information. The best theses used to be selected and published by Dr Webster and Smellie, but I hear nothing of that work of late. Dr Lowder[6] of this place being dead a fine collection of books to be disposed of, but probably in London. I miss him much as he and I used to interchange books often. The College and Licenciates[?] tho' learned bodies seem in a torpid state and bring forth nothing collectively tho' some individuals are still active. I hope this will find you and Mrs Woodforde well and am Dr Sir,

yrs assuredly

Mr B. Dawson desires}
his Compliments}

A. Fothergill

I send for yr perusal White on bilious fevers[7] but have not read it. Also Gibbes on Bath water.[8]

[1] Fothergill obviously considered the case to be akin to scurvy, regarded as a disease of the blood in which acidic preparations were called for.

[2] The transcription has 5, but Letter **75** indicates 4, which makes more sense in the light of what follows.

[3] The transcription has 22nd .This must be an error. 6th would make most sense. See letter **75**.

[4] "Some things good, some things bad, some in-between". See also letter **74**.

[5] The 20th volume appeared in 1795 and was continued as *Annals of medicine*. See letter **62**, note 2.

[6] William Lowder died in 1801, see letter **62**.

[7] Possibly, Robert White (?–?), *Serious and impartial inquiries into the causes why a great number of people die of a putrid malignant fever*, London, J. Wilkie, 1778.

[8] George Smith Gibbes, *A treatise on the Bath waters*, Bath, W. Meyler, 1800.

N° 73 **77**

Bath June 11th 1802

Dear Sir,

Yesterday I was favd with yr letter accompanied with Gibbes on Bath water but as White on bilious fever did not accompany it, I presume you had not got thro' it, nor had I read it. When you send next letter or packet will be time enough. If the plan I proposed produce the desired effect of suppressing febrile commotion, and diminishing the pulmony hæmorrhage, I am very glad, but must request you to be on yr guard against every extraordy effort, or even brisk exercise whether on horseback or on foot, and therefore it will behove you also, abstinere a vino et Venere[1] for some weeks to come, and till the ruptured vessel be perfectly conglutinated. To secure wh the medicine and strict regimen shd be rigidly pursued. An epitome of practice drawn fm practical writers who describe facts rather than opinions may be very useful, and still more so cases of diseases with complications militating against the ordinary modes of treatment, wh without previous theory must tend often to embarrass the practitioner, or lead him into dangerous errors such as continually betray themselves in the routine of empirics, or rash half-instructed dabblers in medicine. Juncker's Conspectus Therapiae[2] I have searched for but, as I cannot find it, conclude it must have been packed off long ago with others ejusdem farinæ,[3] the perusal of wh rarely compensates the time and pains. Reading shd be confined to approved authors only. Since Dr Simms dropt the journal and Duncan altered the title etc of the Comments, I have been without any medl journl and therefore want to see some number of medl reviews to determine wh to prefer, and judge of ye merit of late publications. Wishing you and Mrs Woodforde's health and prosperity. I remain

Dear Sir, yrs A. Fothergill

[1] "To abstain from wine and Venus". Not attributable.

[2] Presumably, one of the many editions of Johann Juncker (1679–1759), *Conspectus therapiae generalis, cum notis in materiam medicam tabulis xx methodo Stahliana conscriptus*, Halle, Orphanotropheum, 1725.

[3] "Of the same class of fodder". Not attributable.

N° 76 **78**

Bath Sep[r] 1st 1802

Dear Sir,

Absence from home has caused the present delay in answering y[r] last. Tho' your late silence after such a formidable attack on the lungs gave hopes that the plan I had proposed had in a great measure ans[rd] the intention, yet in a case of such consequence it left an unpleasant doubt w[h] y[r] lett[r] has at length happily dissipated. The progress the complaint has made will, it is hoped, afford a caution in future never to neglect a hæmoptysis however slight. The Med[l] and Chir[l] Rev[s], 7 vols., accompanied y[r] lett[r] and shall be looked over whenever a leisure hour will permit. From a late advertisement f[m] Lackington I thought this was the work that lately dropped, tho' I now perceive another under nearly similar title was meant. The present vols., so far as I can judge, seem carefully executed, and if they endulged essays like the Phys[l] Jour[l] they wou'd not have room to analyze the daily med[l] labours of the press. Murray's Materia Medica[1] I have not seen but believe it a work of merit, as that of Heberdius[2] will undoubtedly be, with all the advantages of festina lente[3] and the repeated reconsiderations of a man far past the grand climacteric. If Burserius rivals van Swieten in ease perspicuity and fidelity, and avails himself of the latest improvements, the work must be highly valuable. How far the young Bruno[4] is equal to a good English version I know not, but this I know, that few of the Scottish writers produce tolerable English at least in the medical line. As you have the prospect of increasing your family I wish your worthy partner a propitious minute, to w[h] her intimate alliance with a physician must not a little contribute by inspiring hope, that anchor of the soul.

Respect[g] M[r] D.'s case, after so long a chasm it is impossible for me to give a decided opinion without a personal interview on so critical a question. That the cause hinted at has retarded progressive recovery is not to be wondered at, and being so contrary to the plan I proposed cou'd not have been foreseen. I wish it had been revealed sooner, to w[h] particular attention wou'd have been given. With best respects to M[rs] Woodforde, D[r] Sir, much yours A. Fothergill

1 Presumably Murray, letter **13**, note 10.

2 No work on materia medica seems to have been produced either, posthumously, by William Heberden, the elder (1710–1801), or by William Heberden, the younger (1767–1845).

3 "Hurry slowly". Old saying.

4 Giovanni Battista Borsieri, *The institutions of the practice of medicine . . . Translated from the Latin by William Cullen Brown*, vol.1, Edinburgh, W. Mudie, 1800. 5 vols., London, T. Cox, 1806. William Cullen Brown was the son of John Brown also known as Bruno.

N° 78 **79**

Bath 7[ber] [September] 4th Sat[y] [1802?][1]

Dear Sir,

Your former with the books arrived safe and my ans[r] with little tracts have been waiting some days for a conveyance, wh now agreeable to yr request occurs in your mention of Mrs Gillum thro' whose hands I forward this with Transactions of London College, 3 vols. Whytt[2] being out will return against you have done with these. The small tract by White, apothy,[3] I thought you had overlooked till at length Dr Gillum[4] sent it home. Dr Williams's little tract[5] was sent me to look over some time ago and is a sensible performance. In haste Dr Sir much yours

A: Fothergill

[1] Saturday was the 4th in 1802.

[2] Presumably one of the many books by Robert Whytt.

[3] Presumably William White (1770–1826), MRCS, surgeon-apothecary to the Bath Infirmary, author of *Observations and experiments on the broad-leaved willow bark*, Bath, S. Hazard, 1798.

[4] Presumably Raphael Gillum (1770–1819?), MD (Edinburgh), who practised in Bath.

[5] Not identified.

No 80 **80**

Bath 8ber [October] 16 S: Morn [1802?][1]

Many thanks, Dear Dr for the fine young leveret you obligingly sent me wh proved very tender and regulated 2 or 3 friends. As we had not the pleasure of yr company to partake we most readily drank yr health. I am much pleased to hear of the increase of yr family and Mrs Woodforde's happy recovery and hope her future progeny will be equally healthy and inherit her firmness of constitution, a blessing wh surpasses wealth and all the accidental gifts of fortune. I cannot but sympathize with yr worthy patient Mr D., and shall be happy when he calls here to reconsider his case and render him all possible service as the hint you mention affords a new key to the treatment. Herewith I forward for yr entertainment 3 new tracts wh you'll please to look over and forward before the end of this month (October) as I must return them to Dr Hawes. I am in no hurry about Medl Transs. With best wishes to you and Mrs Woodforde. I remain, Dear Sir, most sincerely yrs

A. Fothergill

P.S. News just arrived of the death of Dr Ludlow of Corsham[2] fm locked jaw in consequence of a puncture of a thorn; a stout man in his very prime!!!

[1] Saturday was the 16th in 1802.

[2] Daniel Ludlow (1765–1802) MD, MRCS, practised in Corsham, Wiltshire.

No 81 **81**

Bath April 9th 1803

Dear Sir,

Your last letter accompanied by the London Medical Transactions together with the additional N[o] of the Chirurgical and Med[l] Review came safe, and I regret that the task of discharging previous arrears in my correspondence has prevented acknowledging your obliging letter till now. An attack, tho' not violent, of the epidemic catarrh has also contributed to the same end, and obliged me to postpone all engagements that did not appear very urgent. I am now, thank God, tolerably recovered tho' still rather valetudinary and am happy to hear your own health is so perfectly restored, as to be competent to the fatigues of y[r] station in such a sickly season. I am also much pleased to hear of the handsome manner in which you have been elected by the Med[l] Soc[y] in Bolt Court.[1] As Mr D.—our quondam patient has not reappeared I conclude he has been, like many others, beguiled into a belief in some of the speedy and infallible remedies daily obtruded on the credulous multitude. How many victims to modern quackery after being miserably duped may exclaim—"Decipiuntur specie recti."[2] Respecting your important question concerning venesection in the present peripneumonies, I have met with very few that cou'd bear the use of the lancet a second time with impunity. Such seems the nature of the disease impressed by the epidemic constitution that, notwithstanding the flushed countenance and full throbbing pulse and vernal season disposing inflammation, yet it is remarkable (as Huxham long ago observed in a similar epid[c])[3] how suddenly the scene changes, and how unexpectedly a copious bleeding sinks the powers of the system! Some athletic young men used to full diet and robust exercise and periodical venesection are, however, manifest exceptions to the general rule and may perish thro' neglect of venesection in the first stage of the disease, especially where there is a strong tendency to congestion either to the lungs or brain attended with acute fixed pain, orthopnoea, dry skin, delirium etc. In doubtful cases it is a golden rule to bleed with the finger on the pulse, if this rise and grow fuller proceed, but if it sink or falter stop immediately. It is much easier to reduce strength than to gain it. The natural and most favorable crisis in this, as well as the slighter attacks of the disease, as in the general influenza, is a free and copious expectoration, w[h] supersedes bleeding, and most other evacuants. In Paris the epidemic reigned many weeks before it arrived in London and is said to have swept off at least one fourth of those that were seized. Either the disease was more virulent or the treatment injudicious; the great fatality has by some been attributed, and perhaps not unjustly, to profuse venesection w[h] it is hoped, tho' some times abused, yet is seldom carr[d] to so dangerous an excess in this country. Certain physic[s] have run into the opposite extreme, and not only drench their patients with red port by way of prophylactic, but support them, as they call it, thro' the disease by frequent glasses of brandy and even brag of their success in thus carrying them thro' hair breadth escapes!!![4] No wonder, for if they escape, they escape as by fire! Thus the children of Ammon of old were forced to pass thro' the fire to Moloch! "Incidit in Scyllam cupiens vitare Charybdem."[5] But there is no method too preposterous for some men to adopt. Whether this epidemic be contagious or not is a question on w[h], as Sir Roger De Coverley observes,[6] which may be said on both sides. Accordingly the faculty are, and perhaps long will be divided on the subject. As soon as I can find leisure to glance over your numbers, I shall expect entertainment especially from your remarks on Burserius. That you and M[rs] Woodforde may long enjoy uninterrupted health and prosperity is the earnest wish of D[r] Sir, yours etc.

A. Fothergill

P.S. Perhaps you may hear of some place that may suit M[r] Jackson an intelligent young surgeon-apoth[y]. I inclose the two letters partly for your amusement, partly as making weight—now a small parcel.

[1] The Medical Society of London was at Bolt Court.

[2] "We are deceived by a mirage of right". Horace, *Art of poetry*, 25. See also letter **21**.

[3] John Huxham, *An essay on fevers, and their various kinds, as depending on different constitutions of the blood: with dissertations on slow nervous fevers; on putrid, pestilential, spotted fevers; on the small-pox; and on pleurisies and peripneumonies*, London, S. Austen, 1750. Many subsequent editions.

[4] Brandy was regularly employed as a remedy by the Brunonians, the followers of John Brown. See Guenter B. Risse, 'Brunonian therapeutics: new wine in old bottles?', in W. F. Bynum and Roy Porter (eds.), *Brunonianism in Britain and Europe*, London, Wellcome Institute for the History of Medicine, 1998, *Medical History* Supplement No. 8, pp. 46–62.

[5] "He crashes into Scylla while wishing to avoid Charybdis". Philip Gaultier de Lille.

[6] Sir Roger De Coverley, a character described by Addison in the *Spectator.*

N[o] 82 **82**

Bath August 10th [1803]

Dear Sir,

A declining state of health of many weeks back since I had the influenza obliges me with the advice of med[l] friends in concurrence with my own opinion to undertake a journey. This and a variety of avocations have deprived me of reading your med[l] journ[l]. I had, however, packed them up ready for Saturday's carrier with many thanks and am sorry they have been so long detained.

Sydenham with a choice few being packed and mailed down. I regret you cannot have the former and that you must not expect this long long time to hear again

from D[r] Sir, y[r] sincere friend

Vale! et cave ut valeas[1] A. Fothergill

N.B. A very urgent message from Frome waits impatiently and forbids more. Best respects to M[rs] Woodforde and all enquiring friends.

[1] Farewell! and take care you keep well". See also letters **31**, **32**, **33**, and **84**.

N[o] 83 **83**

Bristol 7[ber] 7th [September 1803]

D[r] D[r]

Before I embark I cannot let slip the opport[y] (tho' extremely short) of acknowledging your kind and anxious letter, which amidst a crowd of others of similar and friendly import have been pouring in from various quarters, as I foresaw, and therefore wished to avoid the painful task of a formal farewell, and as this resolution has been pursued towards all, none I hope on due consideration will take it amiss. The determination respecting a tour in America and to visit those friends with whom I had these 15 years or upwards maintained a friendly and interesting correspondence, has been ever a favorite wish, and tho' for prudential reasons not publicl^y mentioned, has at length only been accelerated by a declining state of health and the candid opinion of medical friends, of no small experience. I am not the less obliged to you, however, for your kind offer and very affectionate letter. My health I trust (if we arrive safe) will improve, and you must not consider this as a final, only a temporary separation and that, in due time, I flatter myself with the hopes of revisiting my native country and beloved friends. But you and my other friends must not be impatient to hear f^m me, till I have had time to make little excursions where lett^rs are to be delivered, and fix on headquarters. A constitutional state of weak lungs is the source of my complaints but none of the symp^s very severe or very alarming. The vessel, ready to drop down tow^ds King's road, forbids more. Health and prosperity attend you and Mrs Woodforde and all enquiring friends adieu! A. Fothergill

P.S. Y^r books I conclude arrived safe with due thanks, but I regretted as the inn keeper wou'd not receive money in the carrier's absence, Robert was obliged to let 'em go with carriage unpaid.

N° 77 **84**

Bath Mond: 30th Nov.[1]

Dear Sir,

I was favored with your letter yesterday evening and take the earliest opportunity of answering it. Last week I had reconnoitered Milsom and Bond Street and have this morn^g renewed the survey and the following is the result; Edgar buildings quite full. Milsom Street 34, Wests, Milleners, have 2 drawing rooms, 2 attics, 1 dressing room, 1 hall and the use of the kitchen etc. at 4 guineas per week, without linen.

Wm Games, Jeweller, Milsom Street.

1 Back parlour, 2 best bedrooms, 1 garret and hall. 3 Guineas without linen—NB Cannot spare kitchen but will work for a family.

Rummins—12 Bond Street—2 Bedrooms, 2 Servants rooms, 1 sitting room—perhaps 1 more sitting room by Monday next but not certain. 3 Guineas and half including the use of linen.

None will promise without entering immediately, so there is no time to be lost. Cuffs, Druggist, Milsom Street,[2] let since my former inquiry and all upon the alert. From the above y^r friend Mr Bennet will be able to determine and a line may be directed, or perhaps better to the parties themselves, the sooner the better. Any luggage sent here shall be taken care of, and I shall be glad to render you or y^r friends any acceptable service I can. Please to remember me to my worthy quondam Patient Revd Mr Moss, to whom I wish success and that you may have the pleasure of restoring him and that every thing may conspire to render y^{r} approaching happiness complete. Vale! et cave ut valeas![3] Adieu

A: Fothergill

[1] This letter bears no obvious relation to the rest of the correspondence. It does seem to have been from Fothergill, and probably from the period before he left for Philadelphia. We have included it here before the letters from Philadelphia for completeness.

[2] Presumably John Cuff (1780?–1809?), chemist and druggist, located in Milsom Street, Bath.

[3] "Farewell! and take care you keep well". See letters **31**, **32**, **33**, and **82**.

N° 84 **85**

{Philadelphia July 4th 1809
{M^{r} J^{n} Warden's Merch[ant?].

Before me, dear D^{r}, is y^{r} truly grateful and affectionate letter of April 30 w^{h} I received yesterday and gladly embrace this opportunity of answering it immediately under cover to my friend Mr Vanderhoist, American Consul at Bristol. But as Mr Warden's ship is ready to sail, brief I must be. Y^{r} long silence made me think you remiss, and one letter of mine having not reached you probably impressed you with a similar suspicion of my tardiness. To maintain a regular correspondence at the distance of 3500 miles in such critical times is indeed no easy task. For the late long interruption, tho' we lament it, we can only mutually plead "Veniam petimus[que] dabimusque vicissim."[1] From a polite and friendly letter with w^{h} the new President (Mr Madison)[2] lately honored me I have reason to hope the late national animosities will be amicably adjusted, and a friendly intercourse with Great Brit^{n} revived, in spite of the Corsican tyrant and his intriguing emissaries.[3] The Bristol trade to this country has long been engaged by Liverpool so that a ship to Bristol is become a "rara avis".[4] Hence the cheapest part of conveyance is in a manner lost. Your letter tho' single bears the British postmark of 2/7 w^{h} seems exhorbitant, by a Bristol ship wou'd only have been a mere trifle. The Lond^{n} Post Office I understand will not now receive a letter for America without insisting first of all on the full pay for the whole way—a grievance w^{h} requires redress. The pleasure I received from y^{r} lett^{r} was alloyed by the difficulty of deciphering several words, especially of names of authors w^{h} after repeated trials I was obliged to give up. To prevent this in future only keep y^{r} right elbow nearer the breast and make the lett^{rs} more close and compact resembling an Italian hand. What wits may ensue from mistaking the letters and recipes of a physician! "Felix quem faciunt aliena pericula cautam."[5]

Books as well as letters have been occasionally captured in their transit to America, as our Philosoph^{l} Society as well as individuals have witnessed. In the United States are many colleges—the University of Philadelphia is the chief for medical degrees—require 2 years residence and by a new rule the candidate is not obliged to publish his thesis unless he chooses to do it. In April last I saw 62 diplomas conferr'd. Theses and examinations all in English. To obtain a degree a pupil must attend all the professors and pay to each 20 ^{Dolls}—4$^{£}$ 10^{s} 0^{d}.[6] Here all the branches of medicine are taught and few students go to Edin^{r}

—Dr Woodhouse profess^{r} of chem^{y}[7] died last week, apoplectic in his 39 year. 3 candidates offer for the chair. Last year has been fatal to many med^{l} men. Among whom I have lost my invaluable ever to be lamented friend Dr Hawes! whose death is an irreparable loss to the Humane Society and produces a chasm in society. "Semper honos nomenque tuum laudesque manebunt."[8] Dr J. R. Coxe has lately published the 1st American Dispensatory[9] being an improved edit^{n} of the last Edin^{r} accommodated to the U.S.—the work is judiciously executed, a little vol. called Conversations in Chemistry by a Lady,[10] is a valuable compendium, concise and perspicuous. Here and in the other great cities the booksellers are continually reprinting the best English authors on various subjects and justly complain of the exhorbitant price of British books. Pitt's accursed tax on paper became a grievous tax on literature—for this and his tax on income his memory will long be held in execration.[11] What is now become of his vain boasting? "Restitution for the past and indemnity for the future." What a horrible scene lately exhibited at Shuckbro hall!

Today, 4 July, is the Anniversary of American Independence, almost the only festival celebrated by America. The military in new regimentals fire in platoons. Cincinnatæ[12] and other companies dine in public, drink patriotic toasts under the sound of cannon and martial airs. Old and young keep the festival and pay honour to the celebrity, Jud[g]e [?] Smith urges me to see a balloon launched—and fireworks w^{h} are to crown the evening. The federalists and democrats on this day show their mutual repulsion, and keep at a respectful distance from one another.

A steam boat, w^{h} is really a novel undertaking, conveys persons as a regular packet boat between New York and Albany[13]—another is just launched at Philad^{a} and is to ply in the river Delaware—a noble tide water a mile broad.[14] In the United States are found various drugs, fossils, pit coal and almost all the metals and semimetals. Bones of the huge mammoth are found in various states and of another large nondescript animal long extinct. At the Woodlands, the beautiful seat of A. Hamilton[15] esq^{r} where I sometimes dine, is a rare collection of exotic plants brought from all parts of the world, superior to any collection I ever saw, except the royal gardens at Kew and Paris. In Philad^{a} Mr Peale's museum[16] presents a wonderful assemblage of articles in the vegetable and mineral kingdoms. In one of the rooms is the skeleton of an elephant, of a mammoth and of a mouse. In another the portraits of all eminent characters who figure in and since the revolution all executed by Mr Peale and the whole museum formed by him. Sydenham you'll recollect has more than once been translated with notes etc. a new version wou'd cost much money time and patience, for the sake of small honor and less profit, nay rather for certain loss. "Your ardent endeavour to discharge the duties of your station skillfully and conscientiously" is the surest way to merit fame and fortune, and to obtain what is still much better—peace of mind and contentment which the world cannot give. Beware of engaging in expensive speculations, increasing practice and increasing family will be sufficient to occupy all your time and no small portion of y^{r} gains. Emancipated from the toils of the profession with a comfortable competency and my 2 English serv^{nts} who are still with me I live much at my ease. Having travelled and tolerably satisfied my curiosity with American scenery I wait only the return of general peace to revisit my native country. My respects [to] Mrs Woodforde. Also to Mr Frowd whose letter I rec^{d} 10th June and will ans^{r} the first opportunity. I have barely room to add D^{r} D^{r} sincerely and affectionately yours

A. Fothergill

[1] "We seek lenient judgement and will give it in return". Horace, *Art of poetry*, 11.

[2] James Madison (1751–1836) was elected President of the United States on 7 December 1808 and was inaugurated on 4 March 1809.

[3] President Thomas Jefferson signed the Non-Intercourse Act on 1 March 1809, which forbade all overseas commerce with Great Britain and France. On 19 April 1809, President James Madison issued a proclamation reinstituting trade with Great Britain, thus suspending the Non-Intercourse Act.

[4] "A rare bird". Horace, *Satires*, 2.2.26; and Juvenal, *Satires*, 6.165.

[5] "Happy is he whom the dangers of others make careful". Not attributable, possibly a proverb.

[6] Twenty dollars would have been the equivalent of five pounds. Four pounds ten shillings equalled eighteen dollars. This is quite a discrepancy but there may be a transcription error. A similar monetary issue arises in letter **20**.

[7] James Woodhouse (1770–1809), professor of chemistry in the University of Pennsylvania from 1795 until his death.

[8] "Your honour and name and praises will remain forever". Virgil, *Ecloques*, 5.78.

[9] Presumably, John Redman Coxe (1773–1864), *The American dispensatory*, Philadelphia 1806.

[10] Presumably one of the many editions of Jane Marcet (1769–1858), *Conversations on chemistry; in which the elements of that science are familiarly explained and illustrated by experiments and plates*, Philadelphia, James Humphrey on Change Walk, 1806.

[11] Reference to taxes introduced by William Pitt, the younger (1759–1806).

[12] Veterans of the War of American Independence.

[13] *The North River Steamboat* (its name was later changed to *The Clermont*) was inaugurated on 17–21 August 1807. The trip took thirty-two hours from New York City to Albany. The steamboat was designed by Robert Fulton with financial backing from Robert R. Livingston.

[14] The *Phoenix*, a seaworthy steamboat designed by John Stevens, operated on the Delaware River for six years beginning in June 1809.

[15] Alexander Hamilton (1755–1804), archetypal Federalist, Secretary of the Treasury (1789–1795) under President George Washington (1789–1797).

[16] Charles Willson Peale (1741–1827), portrait painter and naturalist, established a museum in the State House of Pennsylvania (Independence Hall), Philadelphia. Rembrandt Peale (1778–1860), Charles's son, was the author of *Account of the skeleton of the mammoth, a non-descript carnivorous animal of immense size, found in America*, London, E. Lawrence, 1802. Presumably the one on display.

N° 85 **86**

Philadelphia March 13th 1810

Dr Dr,

Before me is your very obliging letter of Novr 15th arrived 3 days ago, wh I take the earliest opportunity of acknowledging by the British packet via Falmouth, the only conveyance on wh we can rely and, if war should ensue, (wh heaven avert), that will cease, and we foreigners may perhaps be compelled to decamp.[1] Such is the critical situation of affairs in wh national discord has plunged us. As yours has been 4 months on its passage you must not be impatient if this should not reach you till after midsummer. We have 100 miles land carriage to New York where the packets rendezvous and above 3000 more to Falmouth across the great Atlantic, yet by that noble discovery, the invention of letters and of the magnetic needle, friends are enabled to maintain a social intercourse from pole to pole. Without this heart-consoling resource, absence fm those we hold most dear wou'd be almost insupportable. Our great cities last season happily escaped the malignant fever excepting a few sporadic cases here and at New York, tho' Brooklin a large village separated from New York only by the river was grievously infested. In Connecticut to the N.E. a malignant typhus (called spotted fever) has repeatedly appeared and tho' circumscribed by narrow bounds, carried off many within a few days, often within 36 or 48 hours from the attack! Medical consultations have been held and various conjectures formed, but the malady triumphed over every mode of treatment as in the terrible epid^{l} yellow fever of 1793 and 1798.

In a land of liberty and equality a strict medical police can seldom be duly enforced, all are anxious to relieve if sick, but such intercourse spreads the contagion and, when the disease has spent itself, dormant germs lurk in clothes and utensils, like smother'd embers till favorable circumstances conspire to renew their activity while perhaps a majority of practitioners deride all suspicion of contagion. "No such thing now as a contagious disease except the smallpox and itch and they are not contagious only infectious." Oh rare logic—what it is to be learned? Dr Caldwell,[2] a quondam pupil of Dr Rush, in a course of lectures combats his præceptor's doctrines and some of his pupils are so sanguine as to think he bids fair to diminish the splendor of the rush light, and will soon become a star of the first magnitude. They will next exult with Horace.

"Micat inter omnes/
. . . velut inter ignes /luna minores."[3]

I feel for the worthy ancient painstaking professor who with all his eccentricities is certainly a man of science and profound research. But novelty often dazzles incompetent judges more than sterling merit. As that great luminary Cullen had his arrogant pupil Brown for a rival—so Rush descending fast in the vale of years, "Sic transit gloria mundi!"[4]

The discarding of Latin enables pupils to march easily thro' 2 courses of lectures and with English examinations and an English thesis, (at their option to publish or not) to mount rapidly to the "summos in medicina honores".[5] The Colleges about to break up, had about 300 pupils this year, what an inundation of graduates will be let loose on the public!!

In Connecticut some time ago fell a shower of meteoric stones like others of the sort, of w^{h} I have a specimen.[6] Here are found most of the metals except tin. Chrome yields a beautiful yellow pigment and bears a high price. Is the author on purgatives Hamilton, the little accoucheur of Edin^{r} tho' perhaps now facile princeps?[7] His works of Dr Hall[8] I hear are commended, but since I dropped practice my ardor for new medical works has given way to other studies of the miscellaneous kind—philosophical, theological, moral, and everything within the range of polite literature. For reading is still my delight which affords a calm serene pleasure superior to all other pursuits. Sometimes I occasionally dip into a medical writer w^{h} falls in my way. For like a true sportsman I still like a crack of the whip. The works w^{h} I have lately been [missing words] and edified were professor Blair's Sermons[9] and Han^{h} Moore's admirable new work on Coelebs[10] in w^{h} excellent characters are drawn con amore with a glowing pencil pattern, worthy imitation. The papers announced Han^{h} M's death tho' I trust she is living[11] to delight and instruct a degenerate age. The above works I earnestly recommend to y^{r} perusal. They come home to men's business and their bosoms and are highly impressive. Selections f^{m} the Gent'^{s} Magazine 3 vols supply many curious and entertaining miscellaneous facts and anecdotes. Dr Stoll[12] and the other med^{l} works may be had of the foreign importers in London more likely than here where foreign journals are served very irregularly and are long behind. Bonaparte you know sinks, burns, and destroys all American ships met with his cruisers. The cortex in rheumatism is not new, was many years ago recommended to my notice by my illustrious namesake and very justly in the chronic state, when protracted by debility. The disease is very prevalent here still more so the phthysis pulmonalis w^{h} in the Bills of Mortality constitutes a 5th if not a 4th of the deaths!! The digitalis tho' rarely equal to cure yet seldom fails to check the hectic fever and to afford a considerable truce is at least an important auxiliary. For "non regredi est progredi".[13]

Medical Ethics I have not seen, but anything from the pen of my excellent friend Percival[14] must be interesting and also from Dr Heberden.[15] Vaccination I flatter myself will still maintain its superiority over inoculation notwithstanding the insidious attacks of its enemies, see the candid report by the Londn College[16] and testimonies fm all parts of the globe. Sydenham as an accurate observer stands unrivaled except by the father of physic, Hippocrates. But beware of his wild theories and his early propensities to the lancet wh he lived to moderate. British constitutions since his time have tended more to laxity and nervous debility to which refined luxury and unnatural modes of life have contributed. We have had a severe winter, my thermr without, on 23 January, stood below zero, the greatest cold I have yet experienced. In the north and northeast parts, 5 or 6 [degrees] lower. Except repeated colds I have reason to be thankful for an improved state of health, my 2 English domestics still with me, all the ingredients of happiness within my reach except a good wife. Tho' an ardent admirer of the incomparable Lucilla yet as she is engaged to the worthy Cælebs and I know not where to find such another. I believe I shall decline matrimony a while longer. You'll please to see our friend Mr Frowd 'ere long and show him this letter to keep him in good humour and to gain time till I can catch a leisure hour to write to him. My best wishes to you and amiable partner Dr Dr yours truly

adieu A. Fothergill

1 President Madison reinstated the Non-Intercourse Act with Great Britain on 9 August 1809.

2 Charles Caldwell (1772–1853), *Medical and physical memoirs, containing . . . the origin and nature of the late pestilential epidemics of the United States*, Philadelphia, T. & W. Bradford, 1801. Caldwell held that yellow fever was of local origin and opposed the view that it was imported from the West Indies, as suggested by the College of Physicians of Philadelphia.

3 "Shines out among all others like the moon among the lesser fires". Horace, *Odes*, 1.12.46–8.

4 "So passes the glory of the world". Anonymous, words spoken at the investiture of the pope.

5 "The highest honours in medicine". See also letter **36**.

6 Presumably this was the meteor that fell on Weston, Connecticut, on 14 December 1807. This marvel was visible over much of New England and New York and became a national sensation.

7 "Easily the foremost". Fothergill confused James Hamilton, senior (1749–1835), a physician, with James Hamilton, the younger (1767–1839), the professor of midwifery at Edinburgh. James Hamilton, senior, published *Observations on the utility and administration of purgative medicines in several diseases*, Edinburgh, J. Simpson, 1805; first American edition from the second Edinburgh edition, Philadelphia, B. Johnson, 1809. James Hamilton, the younger (not related), published various works on midwifery.

8 Unclear reference.

9 Presumably one of the many editions of Hugh Blair, *Sermons*, London, W. Strahan, 1777.

10 Hannah More (1745–1833), *Coelebs in search of a wife. Comprehending observations on domestic habits and manners, religion and morals*, vol. 1, London, T. Cadell & W. Davies, 1808; 2 vols., third edition, London, T. Cadell & W. Davies, 1809.

11 Indeed, she would live twenty-three more years.

12 Presumably, Maximilian Stoll (1742–1788), *Ratio medendi in nosocomio practico Vindobonensi*, 7 vols., Vienna, 1777–90.

13 "Not to go back is to advance".

14 Thomas Percival, *Medical ethics; or, a code of institutes and precepts, adapted to the professional conduct of physicians and surgeons*, London, J. Johnson and R. Bickerstaff, 1803.

15 Probably William Heberden, the younger. Woodforde may have told Fothergill of Heberden's *Oratio Harveiana . . .* 1809, London, J. M'Creery for T. Payne, 1810.

16 Presumably, Royal College of Physicians of London, *Report . . . on vaccination* [London, 1807].

[N°] 88 **87**

Philadelphia Septr 22th 1810

Before me, D^r D^r, is your very grateful and obliging letter of June last, arrived in 2 months and 16 days. In it, I mark with pleasure y^r ripening judgement, unabating ardor and improved style. Every young physician who aims at future excellence ought to attend to the <u>manner</u> as well as the <u>matter</u>, especially if he ever intends to submit his observations to the critical eye of the public. How mortifying it is to observe so great a neglect of this in many modern publications, in other respects very valuable? But a slovenly vulgar style and perplexed manner often tires and disgusts the reader at every step. Under the present heavy expense, postage in England, w^h outweighs the American, tho' sufficiently high, I cannot desire you to write long letters <u>often</u>, w^h might also interfere with y^r laborious engagements, but I wou'd recommend you to take a large sized sheet, and fill it by degrees as reading and interesting occurrences may suggest or supply materials; this wou'd render the work easy and preclude the irksome idea of sitting down to complete a long letter at once, w^h is apt to induce us to procrastinate or perhaps postpone the formidable task altogether. Please always to leave a vacant place for the seal, and before you seal a sea letter secure it first with a wafer, otherwise the marine air acts upon the wax, breaks its texture, and the letter comes open. If you have any friend or correspondent at London, Liverpool, or Bristol, y^r letter clear'd to such a person with a request to forward to Philadelphia or even New York, tho' 100 miles from us, wou'd generally come with more certainty and expedition, unless by some act of insanity the intercourse sh^d again be shut up, of w^h the paper wou'd soon apprise you. Is it not mortifying that England has now been harassed with a war of 18 years and yet remains without the smallest prospect of peace! That the reign of George the 3rd, a pious monarch, sh^d be doom'd to be written in letters of blood! That war sh^d be reduced to a lucrative trade to enrich a few at the expense of millions weighed down with taxes! But a truce to politics—a subject too gloomy to be contemplated.

Dr Rush teaches theory and practice, a Brunonian at bottom but pretends to improve Brown's doctrine, declaims against all nosological systems and particularly Cullen's classification, reduces all diseases to one. Disease, says he, is a unity and there is but one disease—irregular excitement. This advocates re-echo, the pleasing simplicity—but one how delightfully the labor is shortened! If you want to see more, see his essays in 3 or 4 vol^s new edition in London.[1] Morgagni's language is crabbed and obscure—an excellent translation by the late Dr Alexander under the auspices of my worthy patron, the late John Fothergill M.D., is perused with equal profit and far more pleasure, in 2 or 3 vol^s 4to. My copy was left with my books under the care of Mr B. Dawson Bath, and you are welcome to peruse it, but if you have bought the Latin copy, go on with it, it only requires a little more time and patience. Besides it exercises y^r Latinity—a matter of some consequence. German authors are often quoted, but very expensive and often not to be depended on, witness Storck[2] and others full of the marvelous and written <u>ad captandum vulgus</u>[3] or to magnify the author. Beware of purchasing them, many of them soon become dead letter and when sold will not yield half the original price. I hear a Bristol Med^l Review[4] is publishing w^h may give you an insight in foreign med^l works better than the high eulogies of foreign journals. In the Monthly Magazine of Jany and Feby last see how the French extol their authors to curry favor with their despotic emperors, a few standard British writers (evidently their superiors) read with care and well digested will better requite an English physician. System upon system changes, like the fashions, and chameleon like, assume different hues according to the fancy of the author, but facts grounded on experience and stated by authors of known veracity will stand the test of ages, while wild theories and fanciful speculations will vanish like the "baseless fabric of a vision nor leave a wreck behind." Dr Cullen saw their fallacy, and embraced a prudent scepticism. I read most of the late Dr Heberden's Obser^{ns}[5] and his accuracy and integrity may I think be depended on, and demand y^{r} attention. The present fashionable gossamer female clothing urges the consequent catarrh very often into a fatal phthysis, therefore y^{r} caution for Boerhaave about change of clothing in warm days is very just and important. But fashion derides health and reigns with uncontrollable sway. The life of a country physician tho' very laborious, yet that labor gives firmness and elasticity to the frame, and barring colds and accidents, highly contributes to health and longevity. The fatigue sweetens repose, and repose soon repairs the wear and tear of the preceding day, and fits us to encounter the toil of tomorrow with heartfelt alacrity hence "labor ipse voluptas"![6] Experto crede Antonio.[7] After being wet and cold beware of solicitations to drink spirits or strong liquors. Strip off as soon as possible the wet clothes, wash y^{r} skin with cold water and then rub briskly with a coarse towel and even flesh brush. 5 Children already! after the 6th appears—"Festina lente" "nequid nimis,"[8] Voluptates commendat rarior usus.[9] Tho' country practice be very laborious, yet custom and the pressure of the times circumscribe the emoluments, and it is sound policy to render the demands under rather than over the mark. The fees are better in Somersetshire than in Northamptonshire and adjacent counties. I observe that P.S. by our good friend Frowd, and am glad he is so well. You and he will treasure up materials for another welcome letter, and may if you please show him this as a mark of my extensive punctuality, assiduity, [illegible] & loquacity. Commend me to y^{r} better half and accept this token of my high consideration. A. Fothergill.

[1] We have been unable to locate any multivolume edition of any work by Benjamin Rush published in London in this period

[2] Anton Störck (1731–1803), Swabian physician.

[3] "To win over the populace".

[4] Unclear reference, no such review was published.

[5] Possibly, William Heberden, the elder, *Commentarii de morborum historia et curatione. [Ed. by William Heberden, Jnr.]*, London, T. Payne, 1802; or, *Commentaries on the history and cure of diseases. [Tr. by William Heberden, Jnr.]*, London, T. Payne, 1802.

[6] "The toil itself is the pleasure". Not attributable.

[7] "Believe Anthony who has experienced it". Virgil, *Aeneid*, 11.283. Virgil has "Experto credite", Fothergill has adapted this for his own purpose.

[8] "Hurry slowly", "Nothing too much". Old Greek sayings translated into Latin.

[9] "Pleasures are enhanced by less frequent indulgence in them". Juvenal, *Satires*, 11.208.

[N^{o}] 87 **88**

Philadelphia March 14th 1812 [1811?][1]

My D^{r} D^{r},

Y^{r} very obliging letter of Jan 11th is just arrived w^{h} I hasten to ans^{r} by a ship going in ballast to Lond^{n} and can now only return so, as the nonintercourse is again unhappily revived against England but not against France. "Dat veniam corvis vexat censura columbas."[2] The papers here overflow with the King's illness and every ominous occurrence in England, therefore let us not occupy social pages in future with ungrateful political events with which the papers never cease to bore us, copying disasters and groundless rumors even usque ad nauseam.[3] The College lectures are just closed—a very numerous class about 400! So the increase of D^{rs} outstrips if possible the rapid increase of population. The new census of the U.S. is about to appear[4] which will surprise all Europe at the fertility of American females, who far outstrip the noted Mary Tofts the rabbit woman[5] of prolific memory. The hosp^{l} report of last year presents the amazing number of 17 cases [of] vaccination. No vaccine society—the vulgar proclaim the inefficacy of the operation—and so the discovery is left to chance—and to make its way as well as it can. Last week I threw into Pulsons Daily[6]—an earnest and pathetic exhortation to parents, guardians and spouses, to be adopted by the clergy and enforced at baptism, in favor of early vaccination. The clergy, were they so disposed, might greatly promote the salutary discovery and unite in disseminating its benefits by exhortations of this kind from the pulpit. But this like former admonitions are read, the paper thrown by, and the subject forgotten. So daily papers and other weekly ones read by all ranks and degrees w^{h} with weekly political meetings and party cabals are enough to absorb public attention in the thorny gulf of politics. But the evil stops not here. These vehicles of slander calumniate the worthiest characters, engender party spirit and cause federalists to hate democrats and democrats to execrate federalists and produce deadly animosities among families and neighbours, while the boasted freedom of the press degenerates into the most outrageous licentiousness. Instead of composing most strifes and bickerings of different courts it strives to inflame the angry passions and to set nations together by the ears. Thus a 7 years inveterate war seems to have brutalized mankind, and threatens to plunge 'em once more into a state of barbarism. But of this <u>satis superque</u>.[7] Some of the German and foreign professors who had hastily adopted Brown's system, I hear have candidly recanted and given it up as a dangerous and pernicious doctrine. The 2 leading principles excitement and collapse were, I think, well established by my venerable preceptor Dr Cullen, and applicable to a great extent in pathology, but the fanciful system engrafted on this by Brown, with a number of uncouth terms and by pathetical dogmas inapplicable to clinical practice I always thought were built on a sandy foundation, accordingly it seems tottering to its downfall. In D^{r} R[ush]'s works however tho' abounding with wild ideas you'll meet with some useful extracts and practical remarks w^{h} in a long course of lecturing and practice cou'd not fail to occur to a studious and careful observer. But the <u>unity</u> of disease, the <u>fondness for mercury</u> and <u>drastic purgatives</u> and the <u>unbounded use of the lancet</u> even in malignant fevers, you'll compare with what you have heard, read and observed in clinical practice and know how to estimate accordingly. Huxham and other able British practitioners wisely caution against profuse venesection in malignant fevers. The lancet in the hands of a thro' paced[?] bleeder is like the sword in the hands of the executioner. What is it but adding the sword to pestilence!

<u>Iugulare</u> morbum[8] is a Latin expression of a rapid cure, and may be translated to cut the throat of the patient, a tonic w^{h} wou'd spare numerous bleedings and many doses of jalap and calomel. Your remark on the incompetency of upstart lecturers in London and the danger of their misleading pupils, who place implicit faith in doctrines peremptorily

delivered, is perfectly just. In the excellent authors you now study you'll find sound practice grounded on experience. Theories have ever varied and will continue to subvert each other and after reigning a little while be forced to give place to future ones. But established truths will last to the end of time tho' often difficult to be ascertained. Pilate shrewdly asked what is truth? "Opinionem commentam delet dies, naturae judicia confirmat."[9] is a maxim worthy of Dr Bacon.[10] Morgagni in the crabbed original, like Haller, presents a Herculean work, but yr resolution and industry with yr nil tam difficile[11] will in time accomplish it. But let not yr ardor encroach on the hours of rest or prompt you to exhaust too far the sensorial power, to the injury of health, the loss of wh I remember is the loss of every thing valuable. Intense study will, I fear, increase yr constitutional watchfulness in a confirmed habit if too much indulged. The English copy of Morgagni I think quite sufficient and will spare much midnight toil and time spent on obscure intricate passages. Our capricious climate is more variable than the British and exhibits much greater degrees of heat and cold, yet excepting occasional coughs I enjoy good health, for which, and a comfortable independence, I have cause to be very thankful to the supreme dispenser of all good, to whose beneficence we owe all we enjoy here, or hope for hereafter. May He disperse the gathering storm which hangs portentous over our beloved country and humble to the dust the audacious sanguinary tyrant who dares to threaten its destruction! How are the nations under his control and groaning under his iron sceptre to be pitied! How many thousands of helpless innocent families has the unfeeling monster stripped of everything and left to wander in search of bread thro' pillaged country, ruined and almost deserted! Tho' yr letters are very acceptable, yet I cannot, must not, urge you to write often. Postage I find is too expensive for you and franks avail nothing—only take a large sheet, condense under a few heads and fill up at leisure. Multum in parvo and semel in anna.[12] Leave a blank for the seal and wafer sea letters before sealing. With best wishes to you and Mrs Woodforde I remain Dr Dr yr assured friend

A. Fothergill

[1] This must be 1811 because on 2 November 1810 President Madison released a proclamation reopening trade with France but forbidding American trade with Great Britain. Madison was misled by the French; they continued to interfere with neutral American shipping (as Fothergill noted in letter **86**). Madison learned of the French deception in September 1811. Apart from this, the next letter is almost certainly March 1812 and Fothergill would have been unlikely to have written two long letters to Woodforde in the same month.

[2] "The censureship absolves the ravens and falls heavily on the doves". Juvenal, *Satires*, 2.63.

[3] "Right up to nausea".

[4] The third national census was conducted in 1810. The U.S. population had increased by 2 million, or 36.6%, over the population of 1800.

[5] Mary Tofts (1701?–1763) "the rabbit-breeder" of "Godlyman" (Godalming in Surrey). She reportedly gave birth to 15 rabbits in 1726, but this and other marvels proved to be sensational hoaxes.

[6] Presumably, *Pulsons Daily Advertiser* of Philadelphia.

[7] "Enough and more than enough".

[8] Literally, "to cut the throat of the disease".

[9] "Time destroys a concocted opinion but confirms the judgements of nature". Not attributable.

[10] Presumably Francis Bacon.

[11] Fothergill is referring to the proverb cited in full in letters **5**, **13**, and **22**. "There is no difficulty so great ingenuity does not overcome it".

[12] "Much in little and once in a year". Not attributable.

[N^{o}] 86 **89**

Philadelphia March 1812
(Mr John Warden's Ran^{s}: [?] A)

Your kind letter, my dear doctor, I was favour'd with, within these few days (about 2 months from the date) as you express a wish to hear from me soon I take an entire sheet to ans^{r} it by the 1st ship from hence or from New York, for rarely does a Bristol ship appear, Liverpool has nearly the whole trade that yet remains. I am pleased to hear that you and your wife and family are all well. The severe winters here try me with increasing rigour and particularly the late one in w^{h} the mercury more than once has been below zero and even now frequently at 15, with sudden transitions marking, in 24 hours, 25 to 35 degrees! Such are the variations in this capricious climate. The late comet had scarcely disappear'd before another was announced, add to this tempests and shipwrecks have been uncommonly numerous and, to complete the climax, most of our capital cities have been visited by frequent and violent concussions from earthquakes tho' happily very few lives have been lost, nor has England, tho' it is hoped will end in brutum fulmen.[1] Our pacific people think war unnecessary and say let us allow them (as Shakespeare expresses it) to "speak daggers as long as they use none."[2] But time and room are too precious for politics—the papers will give you satis superque.[3] As the language, manners and mode of living so nearly resembles those of England, I never felt any difficulty on those points, but these severe catarrhs I experience every winter more and more, will, I foresee, oblige me to revisit the mild climate of England, and cou'd I meet with an agreeable condition[?] May next and arrange matters to my mind I think I sh^{d} be tempted to risk the voyage hazardous as it is opus plenum [?].[4] But of this I forbear to speak at present. An unexpected event has lately occurr'd w^{h} will derange my plan as to this country. My man, I find, has been married to my housekeeper near 12 months and she is nearly at downlying and if she takes after her mother will have a numerous family. Before this letter was closed bro^{t} to bed of a son hence, they will probably continue in this country and open a boarding house. This they hazard a good prospect for a precarious maintenance. But I still wish them well. To get good white servants here is almost impossible. Plenty of negroes, but generally debauched, idle, drunken and worthless. This is a general evil and wou'd deter me as it has deterred many from keeping house. Proceed we now to the chief objects of y^{r} letter.

Y^{r} remarks on D^{r} R[ush's?] writings are I think very just. The cold affusion is said to have been used here in the hot paroxysm with tolerable success, but is by no means in frequent use, only sponging with vinegar. The varieties of scarlatina are treated commonly with evacuants, venesection, S. Nitre, Camph^{r} and sometimes with Cortex Peruvianus or Rad. Senekæ or Serpentaria somet^{s} with Mercurials and Arsenicals[?].[5] But the disease varies in different seasons and the genus of the epidemic ought to be diligently studied. Of the numerous cases I witnessed in England by far the greater number were aggravated by depletion, but successfully treated with bark, min^{l} acids and warm aromatics, agreeably to my namesake's judicious method.[6] A blister f^{m} ear to ear and antiseptic gargles were highly useful. Also breathing antiseptic vapours and warm pediluvia with mild perspiratives, and this plan I think you'll generally find the safest and that few cases will bear venesection and purging with impunity. In ascites and also in phthysis pulmonalis as well as in the yellow fever (w^{h} Philad^{a} escaped these two last summers) a mercurial salivation is extolled by many. But whether justly and whether the subsequent mercurial effects do not counterbalance the advantages and temporary suspension of the diseases, I must doubt. The digitalis is in these maladies also among the Herculean remedies, but its effects differently reported—"Laudatur ab his culpatur ab illis."[7] Formerly I often found it highly beneficial in pulmon^{y} hæmorrhage preceding phthysis but in a confirmed state of this or of dropsy I consider it rather calculated to suspend and gain time rather than to complete the cure. The manag^{t} of this and many other dangerous med^{s} demands the care and daily attention of an able physician. The consumption according to our weekly bills carries off in the bloom of life at least 1/5 of the whole sum of mortality, and in the eastern and northern states a yet greater proportion. A comparison of this with the English bills may from the result ans^{r} your question. The alkornaque,[8] a root f^{m} South America, has been lately as a specific, and styled the divine alkornaque, under trial, but I hear no authentic proofs of its divine attributes and suspect it to be neither more nor less than a base imposition by some modern Spanish or American quacks. This day died of a purulent consumption terminated by empyema the mistress of this boarding house, aged 31—till the moment of her death she felt no pain in the chest—could sleep on either side, no hectic sweats only flushing at times in one cheek and transient rigors—expectorated phlegm and pus copiously—appetite good—pulse 75 to 80, talked cheerfully—considered herself getting better even this day till at length she calmly expired! Her father died of the same disease, of 7 fine children grown to maturity 6 dropped off successively, and there remains only one son aged 18 who is expected to follow the rest. A striking instance is afforded by this family of the hereditary taint. To watch this and to check it in the bud ought to be the grand object of the physician instead of hunting for specifics to cure confirmed ulcers and tubercles as by magic. In that deplorable stage, nature I know sometimes, as by a miracle, performs the cure, art I believe seldom if ever. To be cured under a particular course of medicine is one thing. To be cured by that medicine is another. How long will the faculty impose on themselves and others by mistaking the non causa pro causa?[9] of w^{h} Morgagni will afford you many notable examples.

Observing y^{r} earnest desire to procure Frank's Epitome[10] I lost no time in making the necessary inquiry of all the principal booksellers here, foreign and domestic, also of some eminent practitioners in hopes of making you a present of y^{r} long'd for darling Frank along with this long letter, but to my grief and disappointment not one of them had ever seen the work. Latin you know is held cheap here and if a Latin author be not translated it is deemed of no note, or worthy importation but to sleep among cobwebs. English and French books alone the order of the day. But I shall still keep an eye to y^{r} request, and if the celebrated Frank can be obtained here you shall still have him. Have you tried Lackington, Callow, or Cadell in London? Theses here are in English and are at the students' option whether or not to publish. Of above 60 graduated last year I did not hear of one being published. This is deemed sound policy both for the professor and the candidates and may save many a secret blush. Formerly some were collected in vols. but the expense 'ere they reached you wou'd overbalance the utility and end in disappointment. The Edin^{r} and Lond^{n} Quarterly Reviews and Monthly Magazine will furnish you with all med^{l} miscellaneous novelties worth attention—also the Med^{l} and Chirurg^{l} Rev^{s}. If you cou'd form a med^{l} club or book society you wou'd get books to read cheaply. Beware of purchasing many books w^{h} are exorbitantly dear and a deadweight when good and will not fetch above 1/3 of the original price. I observe with pleasure our worthy friend Frowd's P.S. to your last lett^{r} and am glad to hear so favorable an acc^{t} of his health. My best respects and I shall be glad to hear of his welfare at all times whether I am here or in England. I am truly sensible of the kindness of all my friends who so earnestly wish for my return and w^{h} entirely accords with my heart's desire, notwithstanding the perilous state of the times. A very extraordinary duel lately happened at Paris. M. de Grandpree jealous of an intrigue by M. Lepike with his mistress sent a challenge to the latter, and it was agreed to settle the combat in 2 balloons with their seconds that day month. Accordingly they ascended their cars loaded with blunderbusses. The multitude assembled expected only a balloon race. At the height of 200 yards M. Lepike fired and missed, immediately after M. Grandpree returned the fire and penetrated his adversary's balloon w^{h} fell and M. Lepike and his second were both dashed to pieces on a house top. M. Grandpree then mounted aloft and descended safe with his second, 7 leagues from the spot of ascension! Madame Blanchard is said since to have met with a fatal accident. The penal laws of Pennsylvania have long been uncommonly mild and now are about to banish all punishment even for murder and to substitute imprisonment for life, hence it is become proverbial that a man must have great interest to get himself hanged! Whether this is not carrying lenity to an excess time will show. But it is urged that capital crimes are now less frequent than under the former sanguinary code. The penal laws of England, it must be confessed, are far too sanguinary and demand a complete revisal. When you see Mr Frowd you are at liberty to communicate as much of this letter as you think meet. Wishing to ans^{r} y^{r} chief inquiries very fully you'll readily excuse my prolixity. With best wishes and respects to M^{rs} W[oodforde] and for y^{r} mutual happiness, I remain D^{r} D^{r} yr assured friend A. F.

P.S. As you say nothing of y^{r} mother [*sic*][11] or brother the painter[12] I doubt whether they are living. A.Fothergill.

[1] "A harmless thunderbolt". Pliny, *Historia naturalis*, 2.43.

[2] "I will speak daggers to her, but use none". *Hamlet*, III. 2. 414. Despite Fothergill's hopes, USA declared war on Britain in June 1812.

[3] "Enough and more than enough". See letter **88**.

[4] "A task full of [?]"

[5] S. Nitre is spirits of nitre; Rad. Senekae refers to Senekar (senegar) root; Serpentaria refers to Serpentaria root (Virginia snake root).

[6] See letter **71**, note 3.

[7] "It is praised by some, and blamed by others". Horace, *Satires*, 1.2.11.

[8] Alcornoque was the name the Spanish colonists gave to certain South American trees which resembled the alcornoque or cork tree of Spain. The alcornoque was exported as a bark not a root. It was used as a febrifuge in intermittent fevers.

[9] "Not-cause for cause".

[10] Presumably one of the many editions of Johann Peter Frank (1745–1821), *De curandis hominum morbis, epitome praelectionibus academicis dicata*, 3 vols., Pavia, B. Comini, 1792–94.

[11] See Introduction, p. xxiii.

[12] Samuel Woodforde, born 29 March 1763, was the youngest of the four children acknowledged by Heighes Woodforde. Samuel became a noted artist and RA, the most eminent member of the Woodforde family at that time, he died in 1817. See R. L. Winstanley, *Quarterly journal of the Parson Woodforde Society*, Spring 1973.

[N°] 89 **90**

Lond: Jany 28th 1813

To D^r W[oodforde] and Mr Frowd,

To you my worthy correspondents I address this letter, to fill up the late chasm in our friendly communications and to resume our easy familiar chit chat upon paper, which distance still deprives us of the pleasure of holding in person. As we meddle not with party politics, nor obnoxious doctrines to church or state, nor the personal character nor private affairs of individuals, our social letters into whatever hands they may chance to fall, cannot be supposed to do much harm to any one. The incidents of our tedious uncomfortable and even perilous passage across the great Atlantic ocean, a voyage of more than 3000 and 30 miles in a crowded and leaky vessel, impaired my health so much that I feel the effects of it to this moment, and tho' after some weeks confinement within doors, I am now in a convalescent state, yet still am weak and unfit to bear fatigue of body or mind. To enter into particulars of that irksome voyage at present wou'd be too tedious and must be postponed to a future communication. In order to make one lett^r ans^r the place of 2 you'll both readily excuse my addressing you conjointly as heretofore, but particularly at this time for reasons already assigned. Altho' then, like a shipwreck'd mariner who has just escaped the perils of the deep, I joyfully hasten to inform you of my safe arrival once more in the metropolis of my native country, w^h places me as it were in the centre of intelligence, of science, of taste, and what is more, restores me to the bosom of my most intimate friends and relatives. Tho' alas many of 'em have been swept away, to my unspeakable regret. But why sh^d we bewail their loss as irreparable? They have indeed retired, but are only gone before. Having discharged the debt of nature w^h we all must pay in our turn, and whether we follow 'em a little sooner or later matters little, provided we one day happily meet again, as it is firmly hoped we shall, on a more friendly shore, and in an incomparably superior state of existence, and supreme felicity, w^h will transcend the utmost pitch that mortals can at present conceive. The present winter thus far has been moderate as to cold, my therm^r—never above 6 degrees under the freezing point, and very little snow or frost till a few days ago and that not severe. But thro' Dec^r—and to Jany 20 most hazy weather and the city enveloped with a thick gloomy fog, shutting out the sun and involving us in a long continued dreary comfortless night, no wonder catarrhs and dysenteric affections have been so prevalent, and w^h I have had my share. Extraordinary gazettes have again and again proclaimed the late victory gained by the Prussians as the most bloody, and most glorious, and most complete of any recorded, at least, in modern history.[1] Yet the expense of our army, navy, and military operations at home and abroad, with a national debt and heavy impending loan together with accumulating taxes hangs like a millstone about the neck of poor Britannia and that of her votaries the poor laborers, manufacturers, and mechanics. While peace stands aloof, and continues to withhold the olive branch from our longing eyes. Tho' our political horizon like that of our atmosphere is still dark and gloomy, yet this ought not to fill us with dismay and cause despondency, since present evils so called may ultimately prove blessings in disguise. Whatever may be the event, let us cheerfully resolve to endure misfortunes we cannot prevent and exert our best endeavours to soften the miseries of the sick the indigent and the afflicted and still cherish the hope of seeing brighter days. In the present chequer'd state of existence men ought not to be so unreasonable as to expect unmixed pleasures, yet are such capricious mortals as to grow peevish, querulous and discontent unless they are perpetually basking in the sunshine of prosperity. May you my good friends reciprocally peruse this letter with mutual satisfaction and be therewith content, may you enjoy as much unmixed pleasure as may be consistent with y[r] real happiness is the wish of y[rs] sincerely

A. Fothergill

[1] Presumably this is a mistake for "Russians", and is a reference to Napoleon's retreat from Moscow.

[N[o]] 90 **91**

Letter 90, and the last from my dear valuable and ever to be revered friend and patron. N: George's Place 16 Blackfriars Road

April 8th 1813

Dear Sir,

Since your long letter of the 1st Instant reached me my complicated infirmities have [illegible] and redoubled upon me as to leave me, as it were, the mere skeleton of my former health and at the same time to divest of their usual interest all worldly objects, even such as have been considered important. A turn in affairs, however extraordinary it may appear, may be intended for a gracious purpose by the Supreme Ruler, to wean the mind at my advanced age from temporary affairs to objects of eternal duration and consequently of sincere and zealous inquiry and in which persons of all ages are deeply interested. If the importance of the object be duly considered the word in your case to which I think you refer more, far more than it deserves.

[Perhaps page(s) missing]

and anticipate c 1000 evils unlikely ever to result from it.

Should any nervous or hypochondriacal patient possibly urge the exercise of your best judgement on this case, what would you say?

Most doctors would laugh outright but this would be rude and inhumane. In a word what say your four very respectable practitioners who doubtless have considered the whole case with deliberation.

Why say they, one and all, continue your [illegible], perhaps the only requisite necessary to be continued.

This was precisely the case for the ailment, which was pain of the testicle seated probably in the cremaster muscle, arising from exposure to mild cold.

dear doctor, you will see how my strangely deranged hand writing betrays my present imbecility of body and mind and consequently how entirely disqualified to give advice on your case or even on my own.

May you and I and all of us under our afflictions learn patience, resignation to the Divine

Will, convinced that the beneficent, Ruler of the Universe will conduct everything for the best though perhaps not precisely as His prejudiced misguided children would wish.

Consult the divine books of Job, Psalms and above all the pre-eminent Gospel, Tracts and Histories.

Our correspondence dear doctor, I foresee must be suspended till brighter days arise.

My best wishes attend you and your fair partner and every branch of your family

A. F. Vale!

The anticipation of an awful change here alluded to, was after occasioned and deprived me of a most valuable, kind, affectionate friend.

92[1]

1

I beg Leave hereby to make my answers to and Reports on the Several Subjects of Inquiry respecting Ilchester Gaol this Day presented to me by the Commissioners appointed by his Majesty's Commission under the great Seal of the united Kingdom of Great Britain and Ireland for the purpose of inquiring into the state of Ilchester Gaol. For the sake of Order and Perspicuity I have deemed it advisable to give my ans^rs^ in Obedience to the Particular Instructions delivered to me by Mr Coles.

1st You are closely to inspect and examine every Part of the Gaol especially as to its Ventilation public and private Apartments to the Culinary and other Offices, to the Infirmary and Surgery for the use of the Sick to the Quality of the Waters consumed in the Gaol and to the Condition of the Drains.

Ansr An Opinion will be given in these several Points by the following Observations.

1st Question—Whether the Height of the Boundary and Inner Walls occasion oppressive Heat or chilling dampness according to the Weather.

2

Ans^r^ I am of Opinion that the Height of the Boundary of the Inner Walls do not prevent a sufficient Ventilation, nor occasion oppressive Heat or unhealthy dampness.—2nd Whether the Air within the Gaol can be considered unwholesome and Conducive to disease.—Ans^r^ Certainly not from the great Attention paid to Cleanliness.

3rd Whether the Apartments are of sufficient size for the Comforts and Health of those who occupy them. Answer—

With the exception of the Debtors dining or Day Rooms (which I think are too small) I am of Opinion the size of all the Rooms, whether dining, sleeping or Cells adapted to both to the Comfort and health of Prisoners, or at least are certainly not likely to impede or injure their Health.—4th Whether the Wash-house and Laundry are or are not well calculated for the Purpose designed.

Ans^r^ They appear to be well fitted to the intended Purpose.

5th Whether the Wood Screens injuriously exclude Light and Air.

3

Ans^r^ I believe they do not.

6th Whether offensive Exhalations are likely to arise either from the Laundry or any other Part of the Gaol.

Ans^{r} I must observe that I perceived offensive Smells proceeding from the Privies, but from no other source.

7th Whether those Rooms that have been used for Infirmaries are sufficiently comfortable for that Purpose.

Ans^{r} The Rooms now appropriated for Infirmaries are in my Judgement unfit for the Purpose, and that the Jail stands in great need of an Infirmary.

8th Whether the Space of Ground allotted for an Infirmary is proper for that Purpose as also the Rooms proposed to be built thereon.

Ans^{r} I judge the space of the Ground intended for an Infirmary and the proposed dimensions of their Rooms both proper and sufficient.

9th Whether any of the Prisoners in the Jail are now or have been labouring under any disease arising from any vitiated Air of their Apartments.

Ans^{r} At this time I believe they are not, but dur=

4

=ing the Epidemic Fever in 1817 I am of opinion that injurious affects did arise from vitiated Air in consequence of the want of an Infirmary.

10th Whether the Courts allotted to Debtors for walking exercise are too limited for health, and whether those parts of it that have been cultivated as a Garden take up the whole of the Sunny parts.

Ans^{r} I believe that no injury whatever can arise from the present cultivated parts.

11th Whether the Chapel is sufficiently ventilated so as to prevent any risk being incurred in breathing polluted air, w^{h} may be occasioned by numerous Congregations, or whether the Chapel can in any, or in what manner be ventilated.

Ans^{r} I do not believe that any certain or positive ill effect can arise to the Prisoners during the short time which they remain in the Chapel, nor do I believe it can be better ventilated. For convenience and comfort however it is certainly too small.

12th Whether the Bathing Tubs used in the Jail are sufficient for the general health of the Prisoners and whether bathing in these Tubs is equally conducive to health as in bathing in either cold or warm Bathes properly constructed, and how often

5

for the necessary health of the Prisoners.

Ans^{r} Two or three thin Slipper Bathes wou'd certainly be better and more convenient than the Tubs in present use. It does not appear necessary to me to use either cold or warm bathing at any stated periods—the customery practice of bathing unclean Prisoners on their admission, being sufficient for the general welfare of the Prison.

13th How often change of Linen should be resorted to amongst the Prisoners as essential to their health.

Ans^{r} In a state of health a change of linen once a week is sufficiently often I consider the present appearance of the Prisoners and their general Health remarkably good.

14th Whether any of the Wells are contaminated by any of the Drains—Whether the Water of the River by rising above the Level of the Drains is likely to occasion any inconvenience either by causing Obstructions, so as to create any deleterious Matter running into the Wells or Otherwise and whether there are any other more Convenient or desirable Spots for digging Wells in the Jail than the present ones.

Ans^{r} For Information on these Points I must refer

6

to the Inquiries and Experiments of Sir G Gibbs and the Surveyors.

15th Whether the space of Ground on which the Jail stands is not sufficiently Capacious for the Health of the Prisoners and whether the present Site is high enough in Point of Salubrity.

Ansr I am of Opinion the present space of Ground is not sufficient and that more is required for the building of an Infirmary but I consider the Site of the Prison very advantageous in Point of Salubrity. The Situation is elevated and remarkably open, not surrounded by Trees, Hills, or any other Object that can impede or prevent a free Circulation of Air.

16th Whether any pernicious Effects are likely to arise from frequent Washing of the Floors and other parts of the Jail.

Ansr A Weekly washing of Floors, which is an established Practice is conducive to the Health of the Prisoners.

The general white washing which is had recourse to four or five times a Year is also well Calculated to purify the Air of the Jail.

For the space of 13 Years there have been 26

7

Deaths in the Jail. The Average Number of Prisoners in the last three Years is as follows, and also the Number of Deaths during the same. In 1818–408, in 1819 [–] 519, in 1820–478. I consider this statement of the mortality determines with Precision the Salubrity of the Jail of Ilchester being thereby Convinced that the number of Deaths among the Prisoners is not greater than what occurs to the same Number and Class of Persons living in their own Habitations.

I have resided 30 Years in the Neighbourhood of Ilchester and can testify that it is generally healthy and not subject to any endemic diseases. The Epidemic Fever of 1817 appeared in the adjacent Towns and Villages many Months before it discovered itself in the Jail and must therefore be Considered as an imparted disease.

The above Report founded on a personal and accurate Inspection and Observation of every external and internal Part of the Jail enables me on deliberate Reflection to affirm that the Situation, discipline and oeconomy of Ilchester Jail are well Calculated not only to preserve but to improve the Health of the Prisoners.

[1] This document is contained in the letterbook. It begins on a new page and is probably in a different hand. See Introduction, p. xxiii.

Appendix[1]

3 Bouverie Street
Fleet Street

Monday Dec[r] 13th [1825]

My Dear Sir

When I had the pleasure of accepting your invitation on Tuesday last to be present at the next meeting of the Linnean Society I had quite forgotten a prior engagement for tomorrow—will you be kind enough therefore to favour me with a few lines, stating whether at a subsequent meeting I can take my seat as a fellow.

I am
My dear Sir
with much respect
A.B. Lambert Esq[r][2]   Yours truly
James Woodforde

[1] See Introduction, p. xvii–xviii.

[2] Aylmer Bourke Lambert (1761–1842), botanist, FRS, and Fellow of the Linnean Society (1788), and vice-president of the society (1796–1842).

Tables

No.	Lett.
1.	1
2.	2
3.	3
4.	5
5.	4
6.	7
7.	6
8.	8
9.	9
10.	10
11.	12
12.	13
13.	11
14.	14
15.	15
16.	16
17.	17
18.	18
19.	19
20.	20
21.	21
22.	23
23.	22
24.	24
25.	26
26.	25
27.	27
28.	75
29.	28
30.	29
31.	30
32.	31
33.	32
34.	33
35.	34
36.	35
37.	38
38.	36
39.	37
40.	39
41.	41
42.	40
43.	42
44.	43
45.	44
46.	46

No.	Lett.
47.	45
48.	88a
49.	48
50.	47
51.	51
52.	49
53.	50
54.	62
55.	54
56.	55
57.	52
58.	53
59.	63
60.	59
61.	61
62.	64
63.	57
64.	58
65.	60
66.	66
67.	56
68.	67
69.	65
70.	72
71.	71
72.	68
73.	69
74.	70
75.	74
76.	79
77.	73
78.	76
79.	78
80.	80
81.	81
82.	82
83.	83
84.	77
85.	84
86.	85
87.	88
88.	87
89.	86
90.	89
91.	90
92.	–

Lett.	No.
1	**1.**
2	**2.**
3	**3.**
4	**5.**
5	**4.**
6	**7.**
7	**6.**
8	**8.**
9	**9.**
10	**10.**
11	**13.**
12	**11.**
13	**12.**
14	**14.**
15	**15.**
16	**16.**
17	**17.**
18	**18.**
19	**19.**
20	**20.**
21	**21.**
22	**23.**
23	**22.**
24	**24.**
25	**26.**
26	**25.**
27	**27.**
28	**29.**
29	**30.**
30	**31.**
31	**32.**
32	**33.**
33	**34.**
34	**35.**
35	**36.**
36	**38.**
37	**39.**
38	**37.**
39	**40.**
40	**42.**
41	**41.**
42	**43.**
43	**44.**
44	**45.**
45	**47.**
46	**46.**

Lett.	No.
47	**50.**
48	**49.**
49	**52.**
50	**53.**
51	**51.**
52	**57.**
53	**58.**
54	**55.**
55	**56.**
56	**67.**
57	**63.**
58	**64.**
59	**60.**
60	**65.**
61	**61.**
62	**54.**
63	**59.**
64	**62.**
65	**69.**
66	**66.**
67	**68.**
68	**72.**
69	**73.**
70	**74.**
71	**71.**
72	**70.**
73	**77.**
74	**75.**
75	**28.**
76	**78.**
77	**84.**
78	**79.**
79	**76.**
80	**80.**
81	**81.**
82	**82.**
83	**83.**
84	**85.**
85	**86.**
87	**88.**
86	**89.**
88	**87.**
88a	**48.**
89	**90.**
90	**91.**
–	**92.**

INDEX